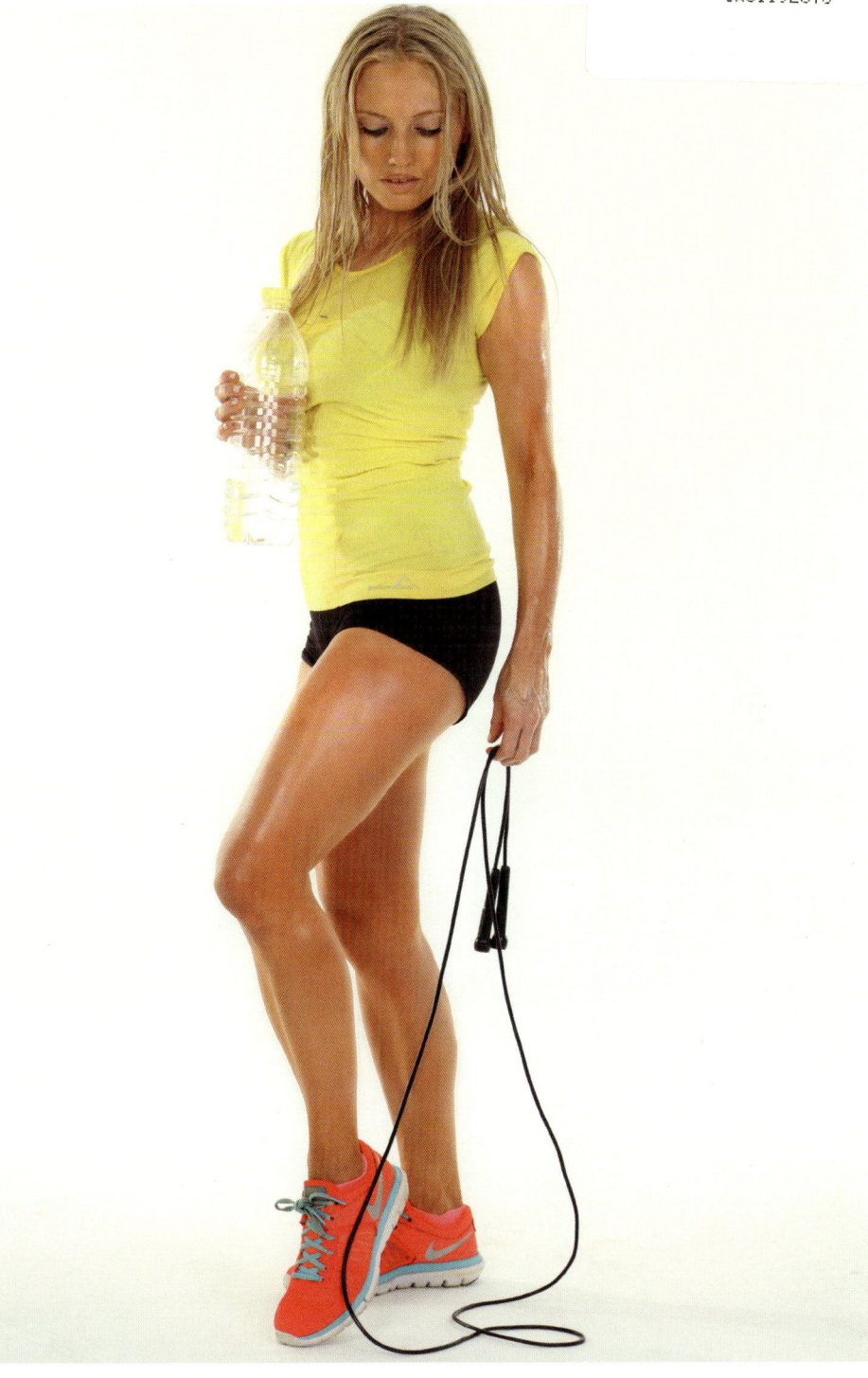

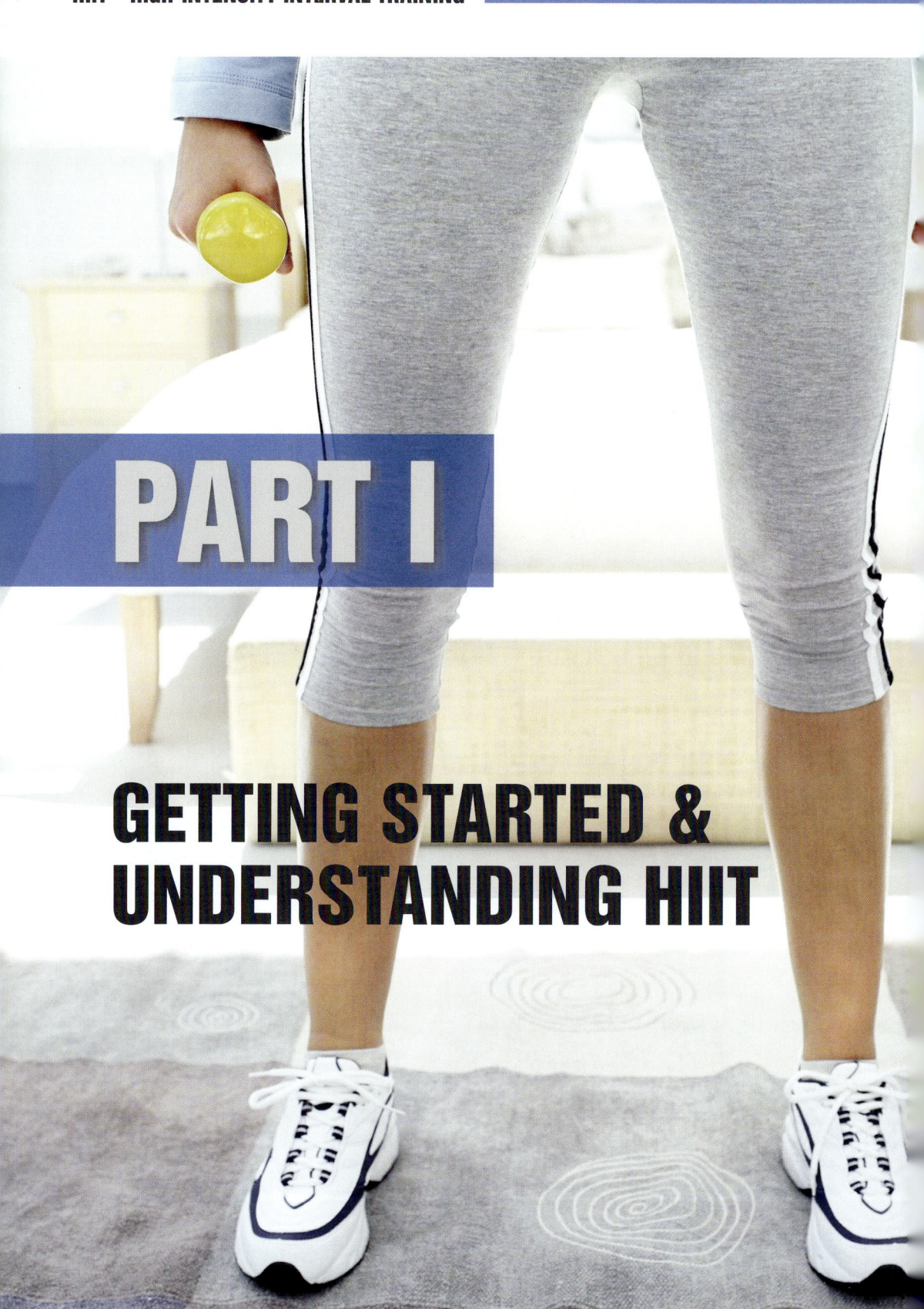

HIIT—HIGH-INTENSITY INTERVAL TRAINING

PART I

GETTING STARTED & UNDERSTANDING HIIT

1 HOW HIIT WORKS

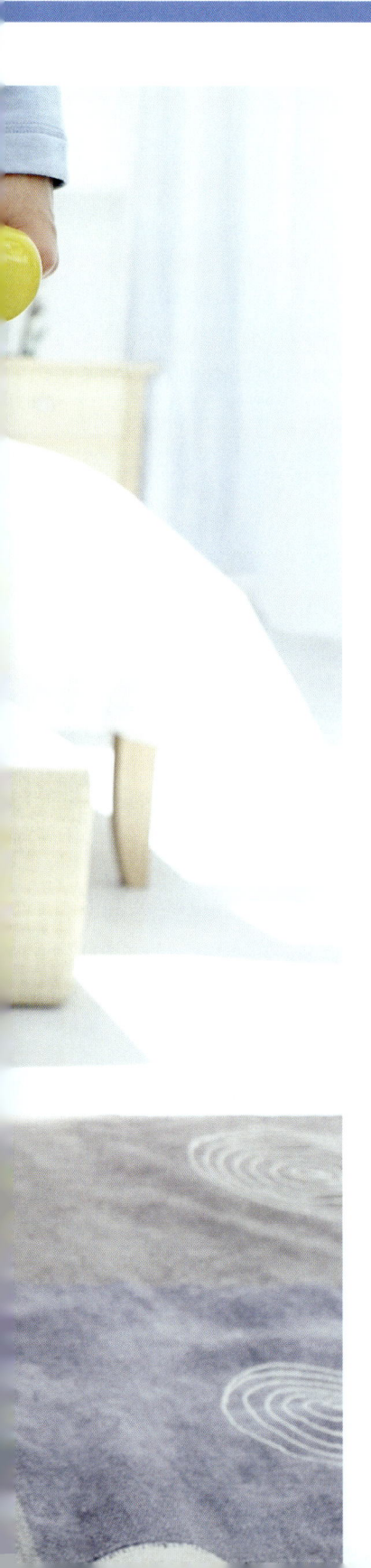

HIIT stands for high-intensity interval training, which is also referred to as high-intensity intermittent exercise, and also sometimes called fast training. This method of training can be applied to any form of fitness, from cycling or swimming to home circuits, and the beauty of it is that it is simple and gets amazing results quickly, saving you time. As intensity is key, the first thing we should look at is a chart you can use to guide and assess your intensity levels known as the Rate of Perceived Exertion scale (or RPE scale). This is one of the best tools you can use for fitness, and we will use this scale throughout the book.

It is based on a scale of 1-10. A rating of 1 would be how you feel when you are sitting, so relaxed and not exerted at all! The other end of the scale would be a level 10, feeling physically exerted to your maximum.

Using this chart allows you to continually assess if you are working out at the right level. We will mainly be working between levels 4 through 7 in the book and will venture to level 8 in only a couple of the workouts. Each workout will reference the RPE level you should be exercising in.

TWO EXAMPLE WORKOUTS

WORKOUT 1: 45-MINUTE POWER WALK

This workout is basically a brisk walk, which, based on the scale of intensity, would be at level 4 (moderate intensity—see chart on p. 33). This pace is maintained for the entire 45 minutes. This is still a very valuable workout with health and fitness benefits.

WORKOUT 2: 15-MINUTE HIIT POWER WALK

This workout would consist of 2 minutes walking at a brisk pace, which on the scale of intensity chart would measure 4.5, then 1 minute walking as fast as you can, pushing the intensity up to level 6 to 7.5. The intensity would be feeling very hard. You repeat this ratio a total of five times, and the benefits are massive. For those short 1-minute intervals you will have pushed yourself to the maximum, and this is how the body gets fitter and stronger, producing amazing results. The other effect of this workout is that you create an EPOC effect, whereas workout 1 does not. More details on EPOC in the next section. So out of the 2 workouts, the one that will burn more fat and have a much bigger impact is workout 2.

PART I | GETTING STARTED & UNDERSTANDING HIIT

BURN MORE FAT IN LESS TIME

If your goal is to burn fat and increase your fitness, then intervals should always be part of your program. Besides being a quick method to getting in a great workout, intervals are extremely effective for transforming your physique. Incorporating intense bursts of high intensity with short recovery segments allows you to keep the workout intensity high while still maintaining good form. The magic of high-intensity interval training lies in its ability to keep you burning fat even after you leave the gym. In short, your body isn't able to bring in enough oxygen during periods of hard work; therefore, you accumulate a "debt" of oxygen that must be repaid post-workout in order to get back to normal. The result—your metabolism is revved up for hours after you have done your workout. Fitness specialists refer to this phenomenon as excess post-exercise oxygen consumption, or EPOC. The great news is that it's very doable to slot these highly effective quick workouts into any busy lifestyle, and this book gives you plenty workouts to choose from. So those days when you are super busy, you can still fit in the quick 5-minute HIIT workout. No matter how booked your diary gets, you can always find the time.

2 HOW YOUR BODY MOVES

A very important aspect of any workout plan is to use as many planes of movement as you can to get great results.

I see so many workouts that only ever focus on one range of movement, and the result of this is overloading center muscle groups, causing injuries, and negatively affecting posture. And if body sculpting and toning is what you want, then using the three ranges is essential; it nips and tucks you in from every angle.

The three planes are:

- Sagittal (which is forward and backward motion); this is the most typically used plane.
- Lateral, also referred to as frontal (which is sideways movement).
- Transverse (which is twisting and rotational movement).

I like to explain to my clients and in my books and apps just how the body works when we are exercising, because I believe the more you understand what you are doing, the more you engage with your workouts.

KNOWLEDGE IS POWER

PART I | GETTING STARTED & UNDERSTANDING HIIT

LET'S LOOK AT THE SAGITTAL PLANE

The sagittal plane is the most common plane of movement that we do not only in exercise, but also in day-to-day life; this is simply moving the body forward or backward.

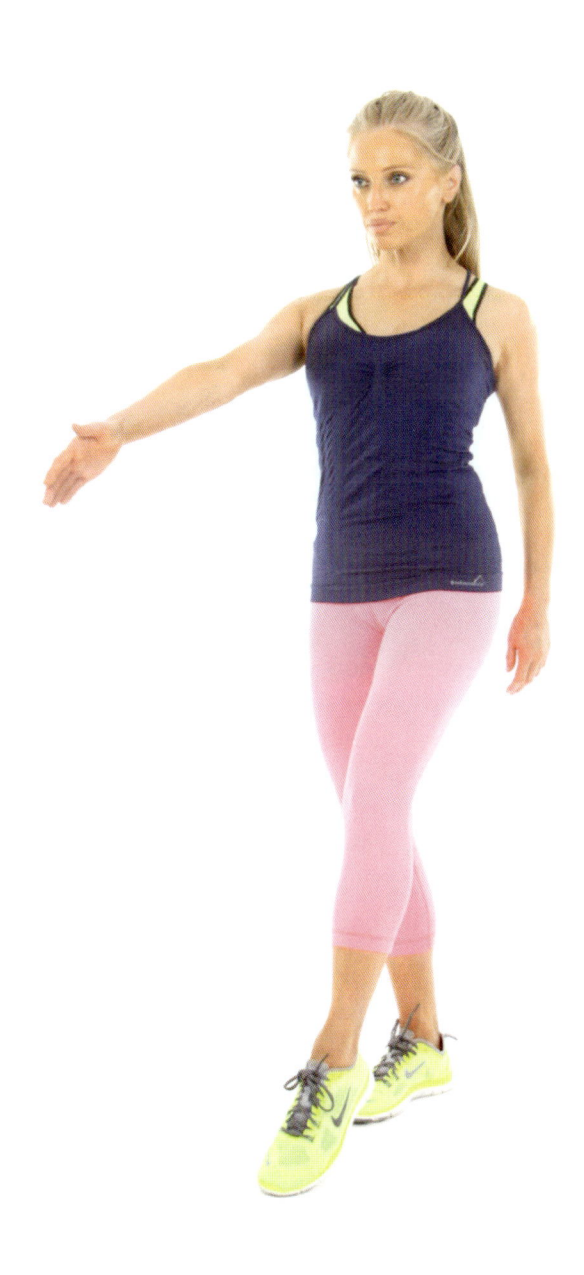

HIIT—HIGH-INTENSITY INTERVAL TRAINING

The following exercises are done in the sagittal plane: walking, running, rowing, cycling, lunges, squats, and push-ups. So if you followed a workout that was just running and then squats and push-ups, you would only ever be working your muscles through the front and back of your body and missing out on all your side muscles.

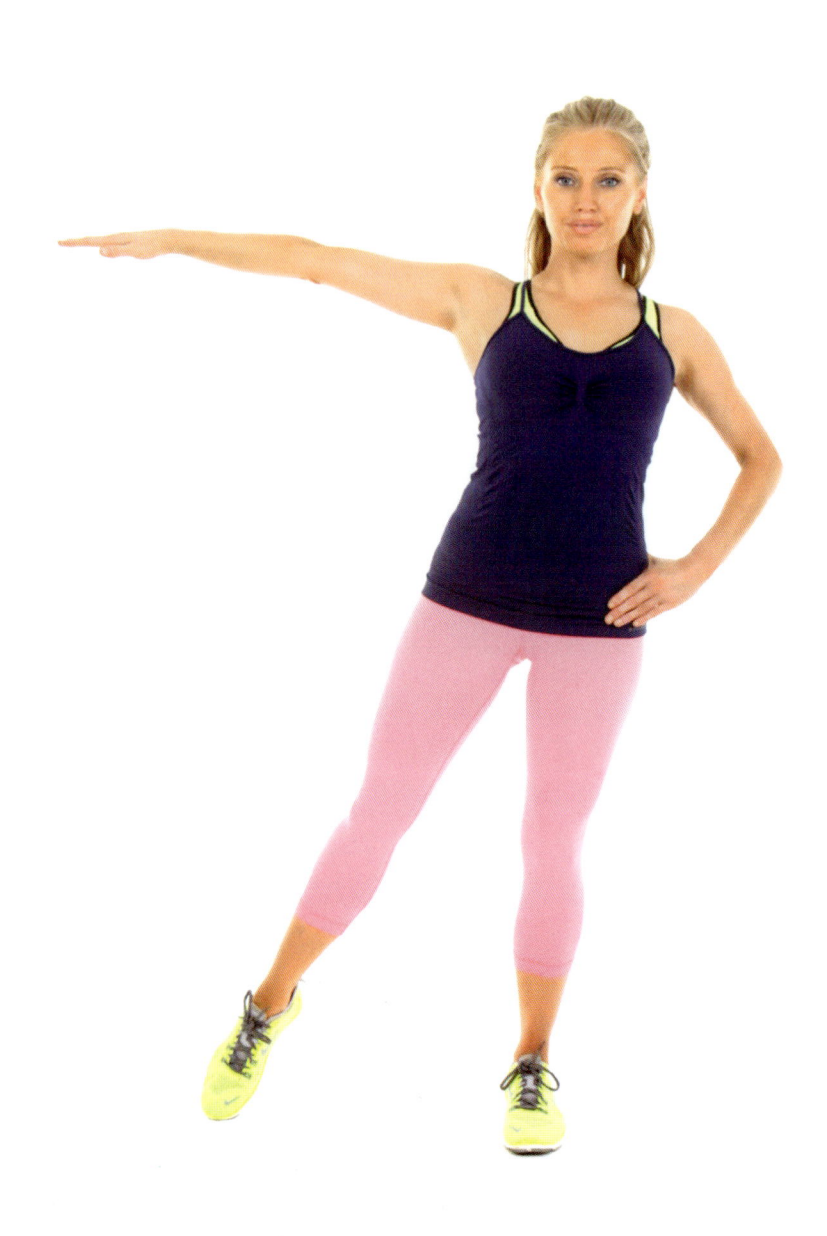

Frontal movement is taking the range of movement out to the side, so this movement would be used a lot in racket sports, where you step out to the side or strike a racket by lifting your arm to the side. This movement is also in exercises such as skater's lunges or the famous star jump. (Used in the HIIT workouts, this is a great lateral movement; in fact, this gem moves through all the ranges.)

Then finally transverse is a rotational move, and good examples of this would be golf, boxing, or certain styles of swimming, such as the breast stroke. And a great example of this as an exercise is the Ab Shaper used in the 7-Minute HIIT Workout (p.64), as this targets those side muscles, your internal and external obliques, that help draw in the waist.

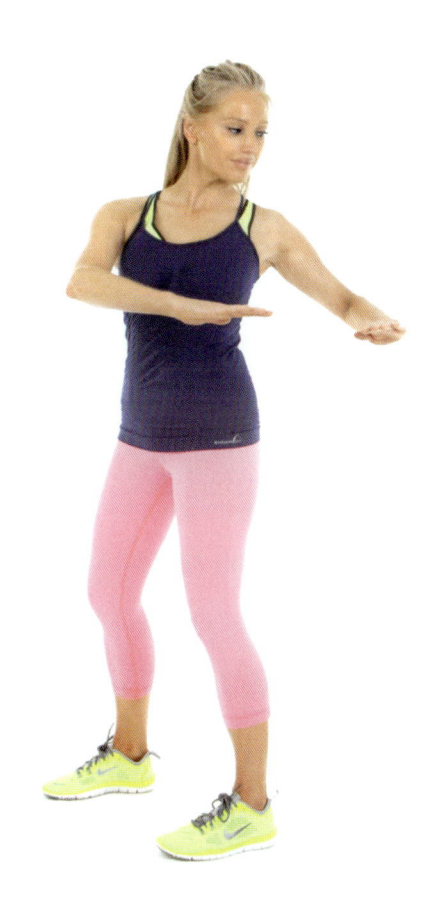

HIIT—HIGH-INTENSITY INTERVAL TRAINING

So whenever you are working out, it is always a good idea to make sure you are using at least two ranges of movement. I have coded all the HIIT workouts in this book so that you know what planes of movement are used.

3 INTENSITY VERSUS DURATION

And the winner is INTENSITY, making HIIT WORKOUTS #1.

Like anything in life, the harder you work, the better the results. A 7-minute home HIIT workout, compared to a 30-minute gentle bike ride in the gym, will gain you so many more benefits, as those short bursts of high intensity are what have the most incredible effect on the following.

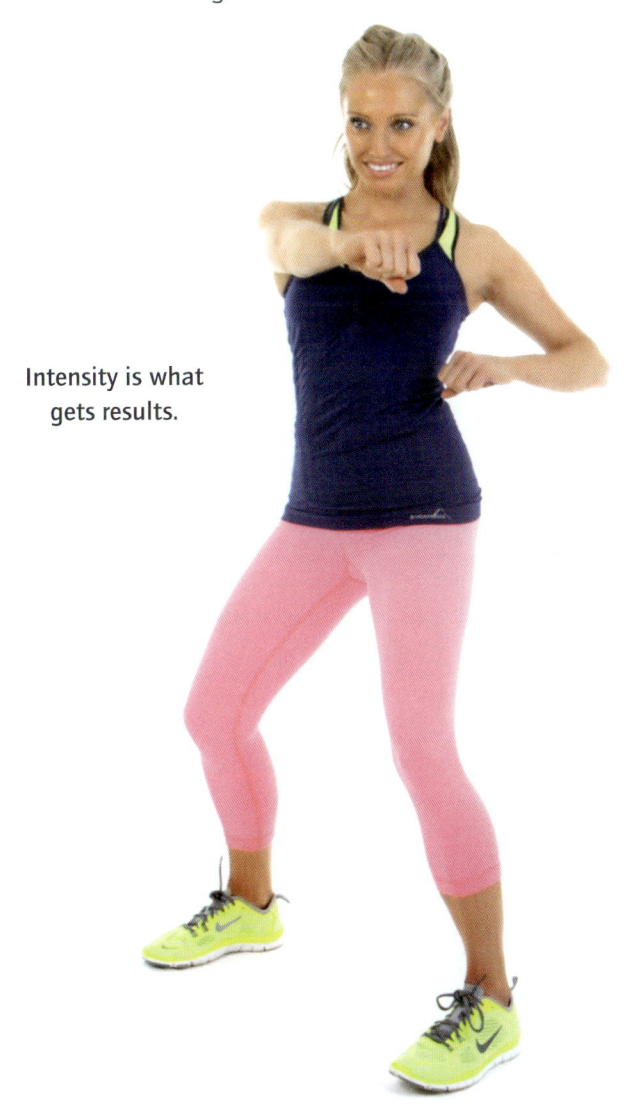

Intensity is what gets results.

HIIT—HIGH-INTENSITY INTERVAL TRAINING

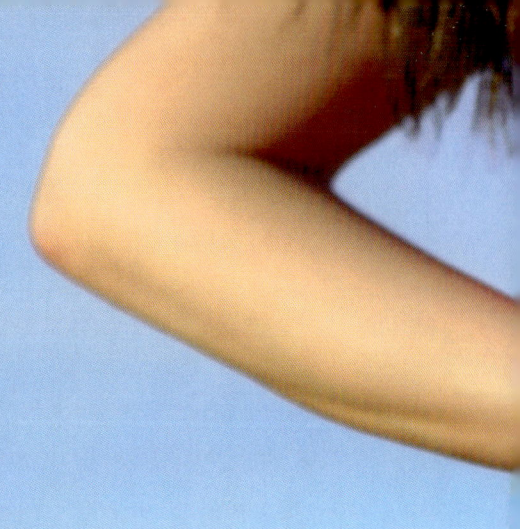

- Increase your body's ability to burn fat
- Improve your cardiovascular health
- Save you time
- Reduce your stress levels
- Able to sustain this workout in your day-to-day life
- Tone all over
- Feel amazing
- Slow down the ageing process
- Improve your general health
- And finally feel full of energy and be glowing with vitality every day
- Oh and did I mention save time?!!

And that is just a few as the list goes on and on..........

PART I | GETTING STARTED & UNDERSTANDING HIIT

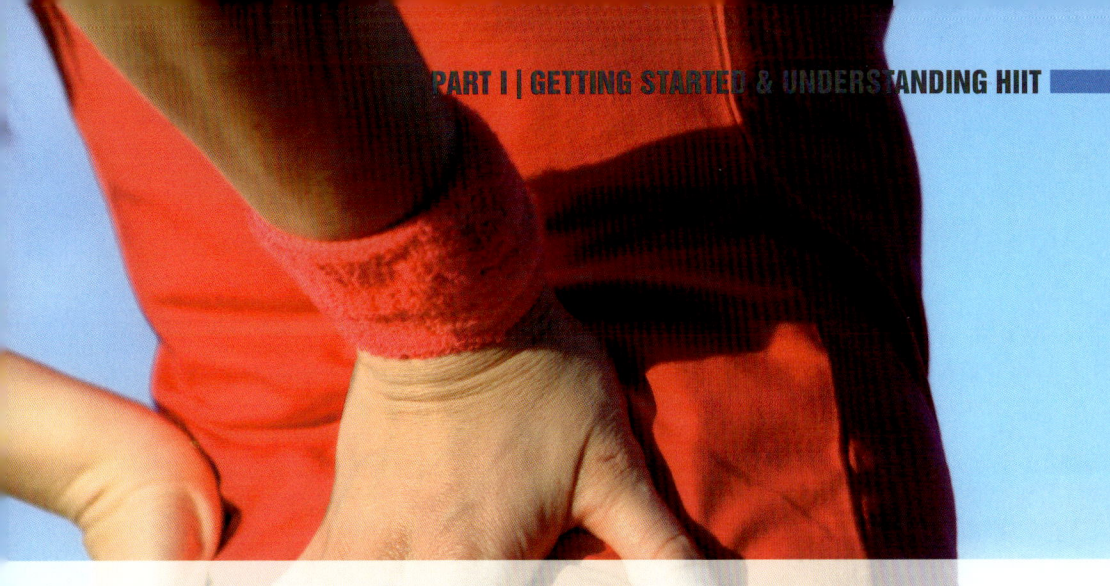

4 FIT TESTS AND RESULTS

RESULTS KEEP YOU MOTIVATED

One of the biggest motivators is seeing results, and with my HIIT book you can expect to see them quickly, not just in your body shape but also in your fitness levels. So I recommend you do the following simple FITNESS TESTS and make a note of either the time or repetitions. You could simply select one, or you may want to do all following five. Every three weeks redo these tests and I can promise you that if you have been doing the workouts you can expect to see amazing results.

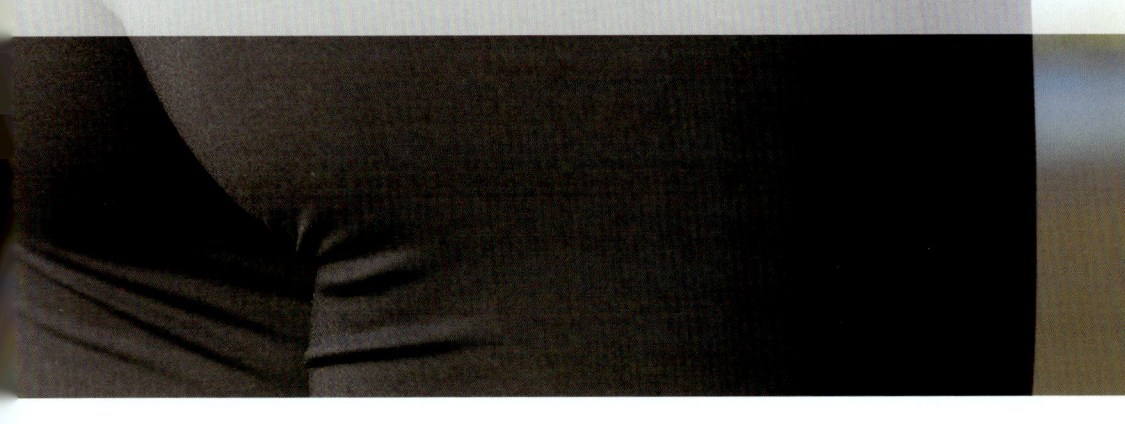

HIIT—HIGH-INTENSITY INTERVAL TRAINING

THE ONE-MILE TEST: RUN OR WALK

For this test you can either run or walk, but simply map out a one-mile route and complete this distance in as fast a time as you can. If you are a complete beginner to exercise, then stick with a walk and just pace yourself. If you are a runner, then run it in your best time.

Date	Time	How You Felt (e.g., exhausted or found it easy)

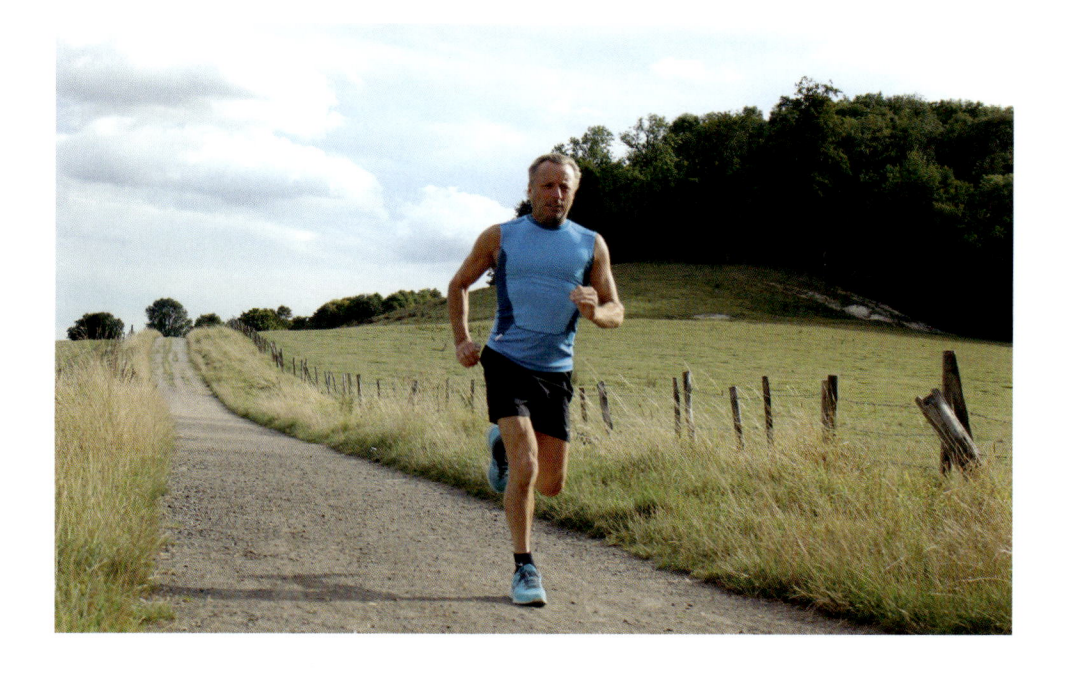

PART I | GETTING STARTED & UNDERSTANDING HIIT

THE UPPER-BODY TEST: PUSH-UPS

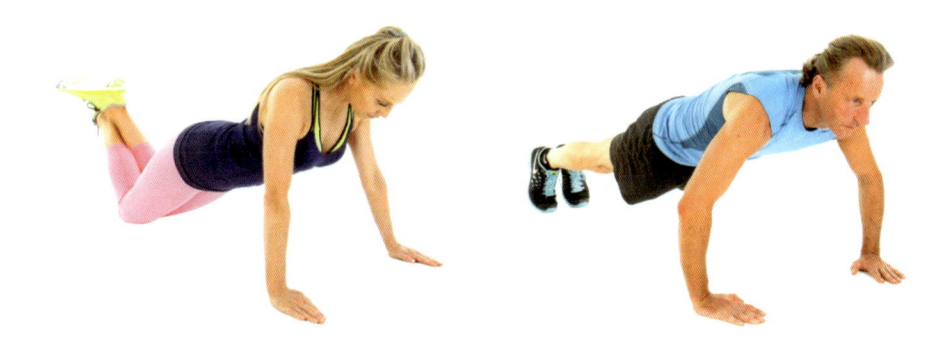

For beginners to intermediate exercisers, perform on your knees. For advanced exercisers, perform full body.

Push-ups are a great way to assess your upper-body strength and endurance. Simply perform as many as you can with good form and make a note of how many you can do. You will be impressed to see that number increase in the space of three weeks.

Date	Amount	How You Felt

HIIT—HIGH-INTENSITY INTERVAL TRAINING

THE LOWER-BODY TEST: WALKING LUNGES

The lower body will very quickly improve in stamina and endurance, and a great way to measure this is by doing the walking lunge test. Simply count how many walking lunges you can do, while still performing them with good technique. Each time you do a workout, you will be increasing and improving your lower-body fitness, and you will be delighted with the increase you see each time you redo the test.

Date	Amount	How You Felt

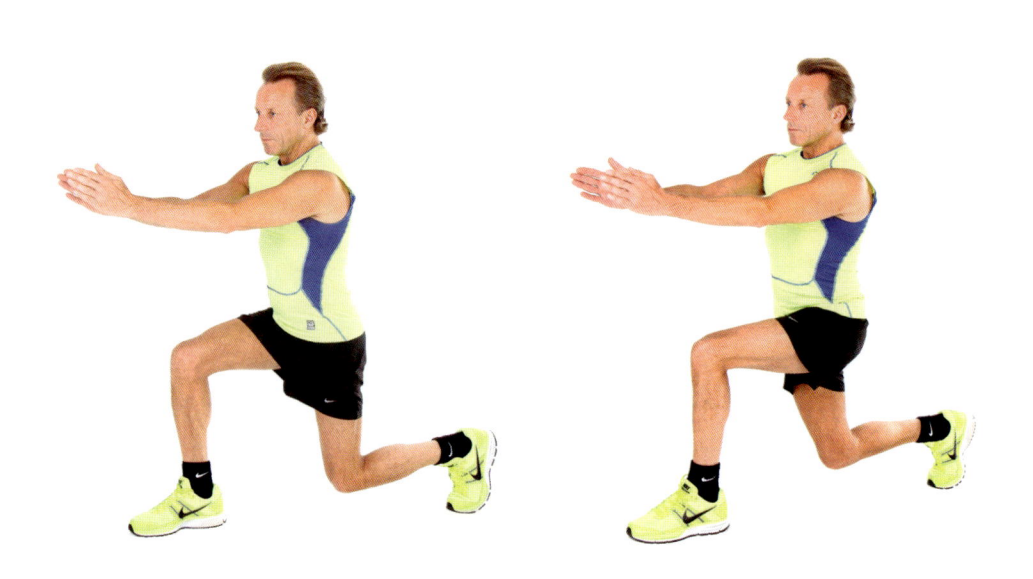

THE HOW YOU FEEL TEST

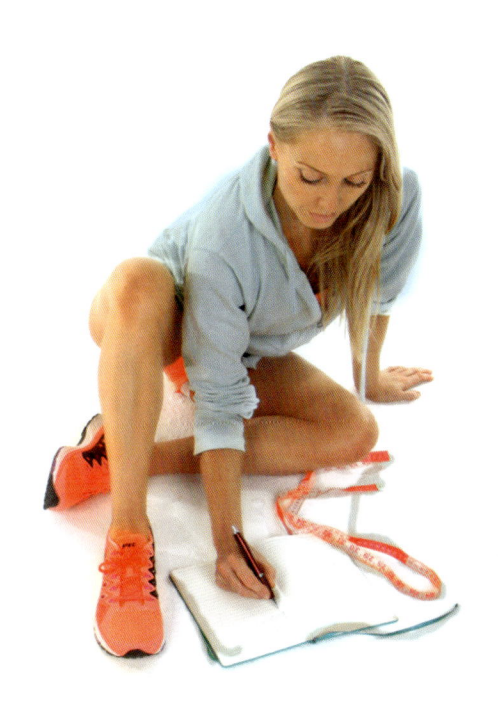

Okay, this one is simply how strong and fit you feel, and for this I suggest we work on a grade system of 1-10, in which 1 is feeling unfit, tired, no energy, overweight; and 10 is feeling fit, strong, energized, toned, and a healthy weight. The great thing with HIIT is that it affects every component of fitness, so you will feel results all over. And trust me, each week you will feel better. Once you start this book, you will never feel below a 7.

Date	How You Feel

HIIT—HIGH-INTENSITY INTERVAL TRAINING

BODY SHAPE AND WEIGHT LOSS

Instead of jumping on the weighing scales, grab a tape measure, because this is the best way to assess fat loss. Remember, all these workouts are designed specifically to melt the fat and tone the muscle, so you will see the inches drop down quickly.

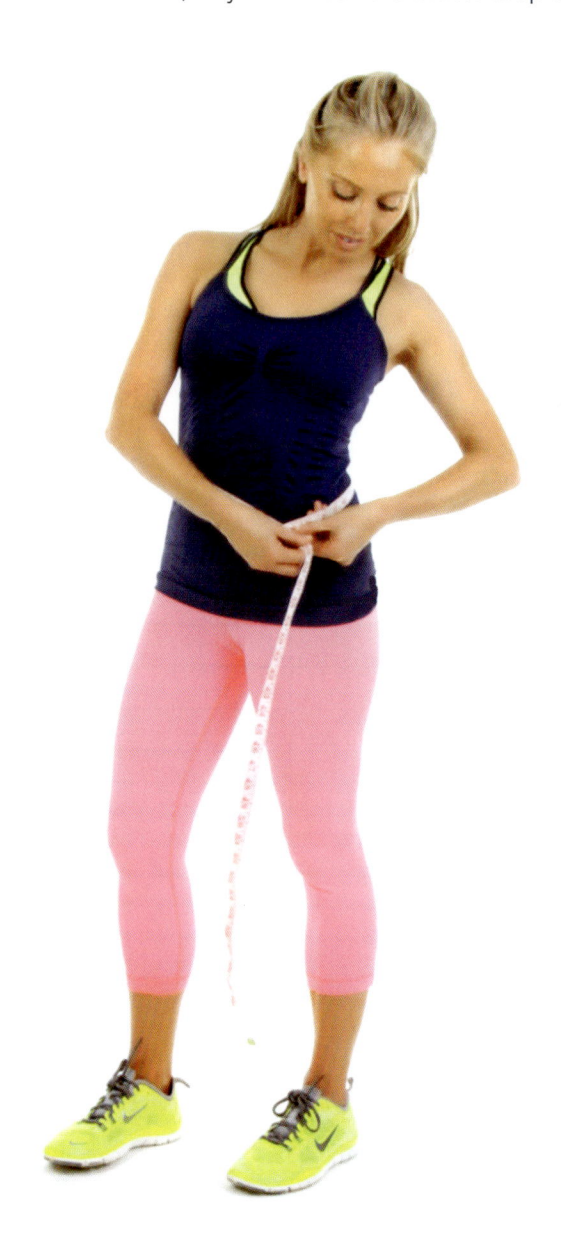

MEASURE

For your waist, always place tape measure around the narrowest part of your waist. For your bottom, measure around your widest point. For your thigh, measure a quarter of the way down, and make sure you always measure the same leg.

Date	Waist	Bottom	Thigh

5 YOUR HIIT KIT LIST

So the great thing with this HIIT book of mine is that most of the workouts don't require any equipment, so all you need to find is time, and that again is less than 15 minutes!

But there are a few things worth investing in! After all, this book is not a fad. It is about a permanent, healthy, fit lifestyle for you to continue. In order of importance, I have listed some good investments for your health and ongoing fitness journey.

SHOES/TRAINERS/SNEAKERS

Whatever your name for these, they are a must, and as most (but not all) of my HIIT workouts have some high-impact moves, it is a good idea to make sure you have a pair of trainers that have a good cushioning sole. This helps reduce any impact and is a good way to help look after your joints. Have a look at the soles of your trainers and make sure they are not to worn out and have plenty of cushioning. Make them a top priority in your closet.

ONE FOR THE GIRLS

Okay, this is a must if we women want to protect our busts! So don't think that a nice, normal bra will do the trick of holding you in place when you are doing the star jumps because it won't. This is why it is important to invest in a good quality sports bra that is the perfect fit and made with quality martial that will keep its strength from wash to wash!

PART I | GETTING STARTED & UNDERSTANDING HIIT

STOPWATCH/TIMER

You may find that your mobile phone has a got a good stopwatch, or you can even find loads of free apps to download with this capability. Stopwatches, however, are so cheap that for very little money this could be a good investment. Then it is a tangible part of your HIIT gym, and, after all, it is all about time.

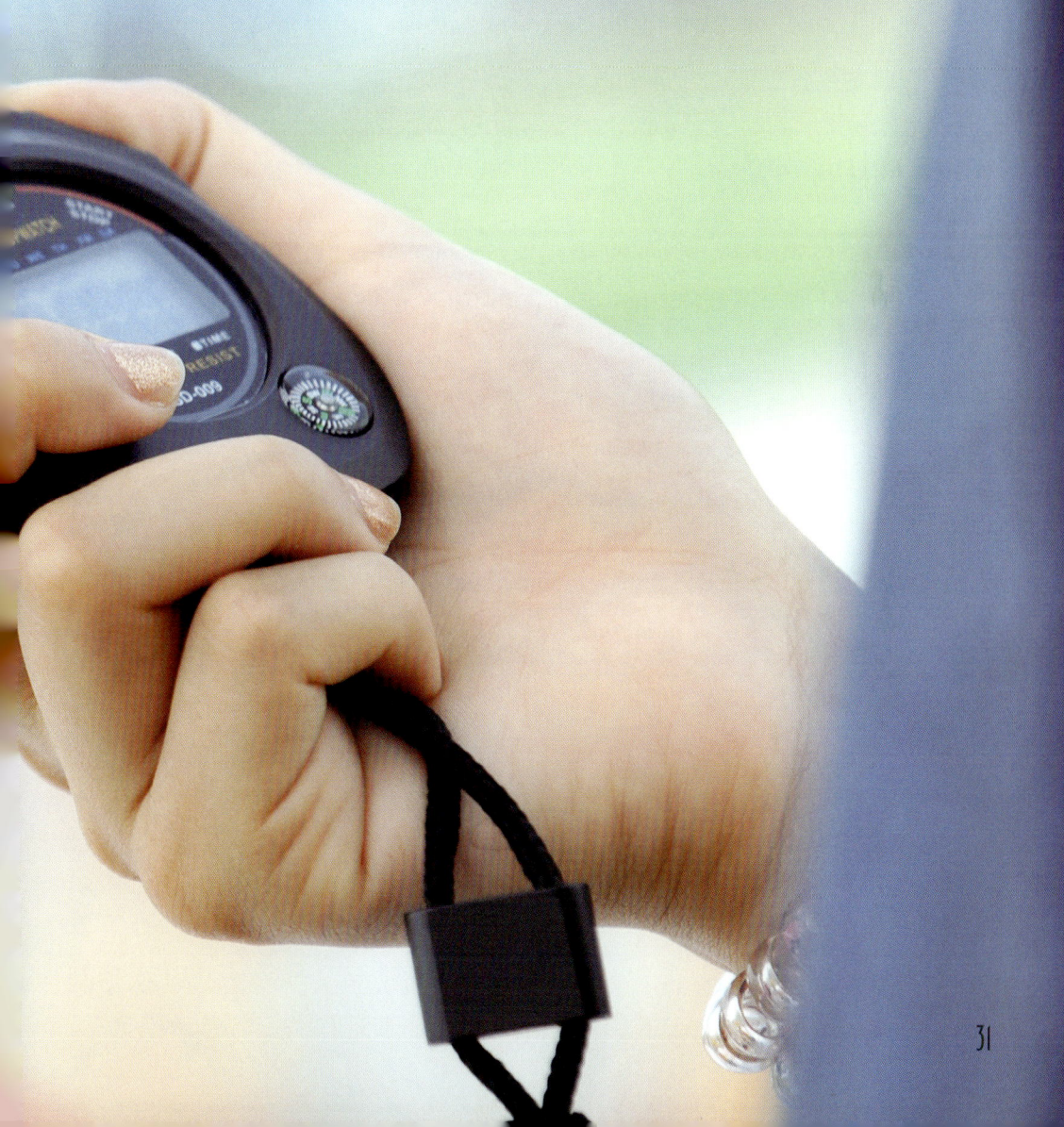

OTHER ITEMS FOR YOUR KIT

For the floor exercises, I recommend a mat, but if you don't have one, a good alternative is to simply use a bath towel.

If you don't have any free weights, you can also use alternatives, such as different sized water bottles. Simply fill the water bottles with sand or even rice (whole grain, of course!).

For a skipping rope, you could again invest in one as they are cheap or make your own using some sturdy rope.

OTHER USEFUL TIPS:

Find a space in the house and allocate that as your gym space. If you can, keep the items in your kit list in this location, ready for when you are inspired to do one of my HIIT workouts.

And, finally, clothing. The most important workout gear from the kit list provided here that made it into the top three of my priority list are the trainers and the sports bra. As for the rest of your workout gear, the most important thing is that you feel comfortable in it, and if you are training outdoors, then go bright so you are always very visible.

PART I | GETTING STARTED & UNDERSTANDING HIIT

6 WORKOUT INTENSITY GUIDE

It is necessary to exercise at a recommended intensity to achieve the benefits of HIIT.

Gauging exercise intensity can be difficult, expensive, and time consuming, yet all you need to do is learn about and adapt one of the best-kept secrets of the fitness world: THE RATE OF PERCEIVED EXERTION SCALE. This RPE scale simply allows you to monitor the level of intensity you are training at so that you can ensure you are working out at the correct intensity for the HIIT workouts.

I suggest you familiarize yourself with this scale because we refer to these levels throughout the book, and each individual workout lists the RPE level you should be training at.

RATE OF PERCEIVED EXERTION SCALE

1	Nothing at all (sitting on the sofa)
2	Very, very light
3	Very light (gentle exercises)
4	Moderate
5	Somewhat hard (feeling a little out of breath)
6	Hard (unable to hold a conversation)
7	Very hard
8	Very, very hard
9	Near exhaustion
10	Maximum

Note: We never need to enter level 9 or above, and exercising at those levels is not recommended.

7 WARM-UP STRETCH AND COOL-DOWN

Before every workout, you should always prepare your body by doing a warm-up. The reason why is that it will help prevent any injuries caused by cold muscles because when they are cold they are less pliable, meaning they are tighter, and you will have a smaller range of movement. When the muscles are warmed up, they become more pliable and less likely to cause injuries, and also they become more flexible so you then have a much fuller range of movement. This means exercise is easier, and you will have a more effective workout.

SO NEVER SKIP ON YOUR WARM-UP AND REMEMBER:

Your warm-up will help you have a more effective workout, help prevent any injuries, and also help mentally prepare you for the workout ahead. Likewise, at the end of every workout, I advise you to spend a minute or so gently marching in place to slowly bring your body back to a pre-exercise state. Then you should always perform all the stretches presented in this book to help repair your muscles after the workout.

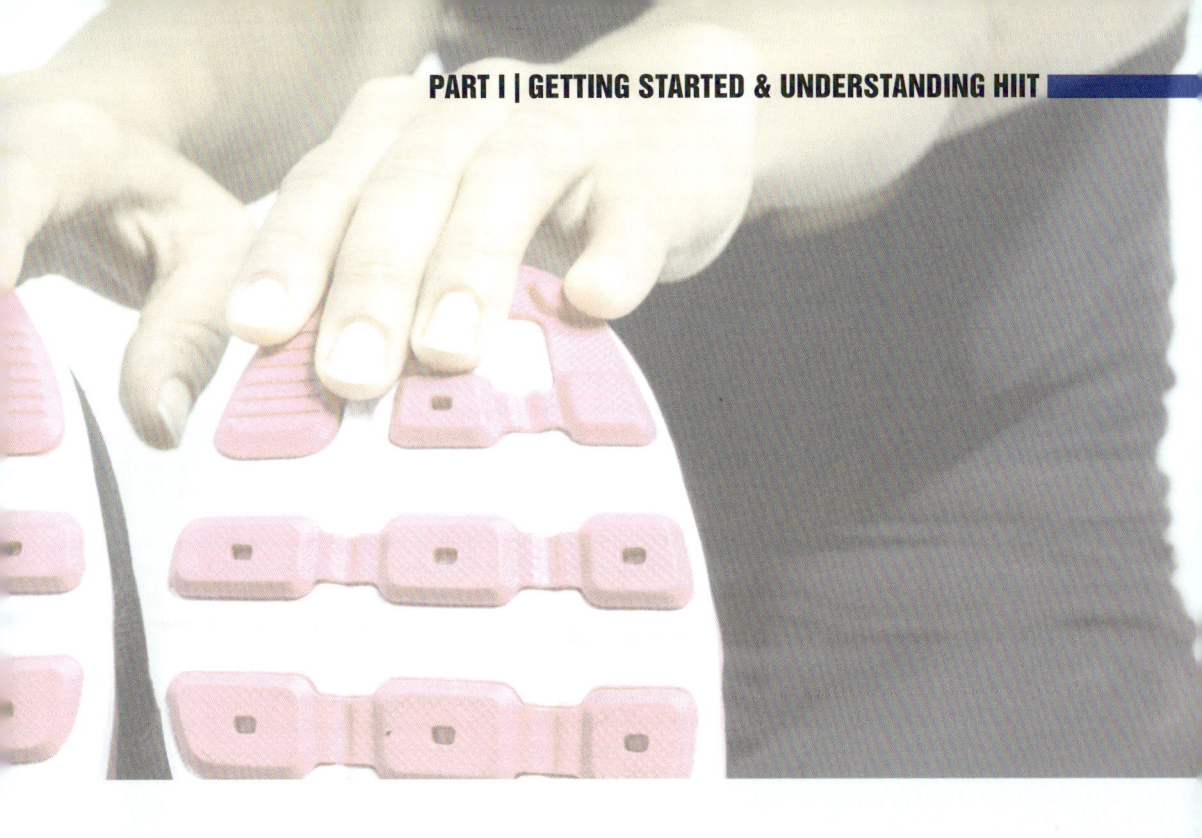

HOW TO WARM-UP:

If you are doing one of my HIIT indoor workouts, then you have two options. You can either simply march in place for a couple of minutes, and after a minute increase the height that you lift your legs as you march and circle your arms out to your sides.

Or, alternatively, you can march up and down the stairs for a couple of minutes.

If you are doing one on my HIIT outdoor workouts, then you can simply walk at a brisk pace for a few minutes.

Once you are warmed up, it's a good idea to stretch your major muscle groups, and this is also essential to do at the end of your workout, because this helps the muscles repair and prevents muscle soreness.

CALF STRETCH

Step back with one leg; keep the back leg straight and the heel down, with both feet pointing forward. Bend the knee of the front leg and place your hands on the bent leg. Feel the stretch in the lower leg that is extended behind. Hold for 10 seconds for your warm-up and 15 seconds for your cool-down.

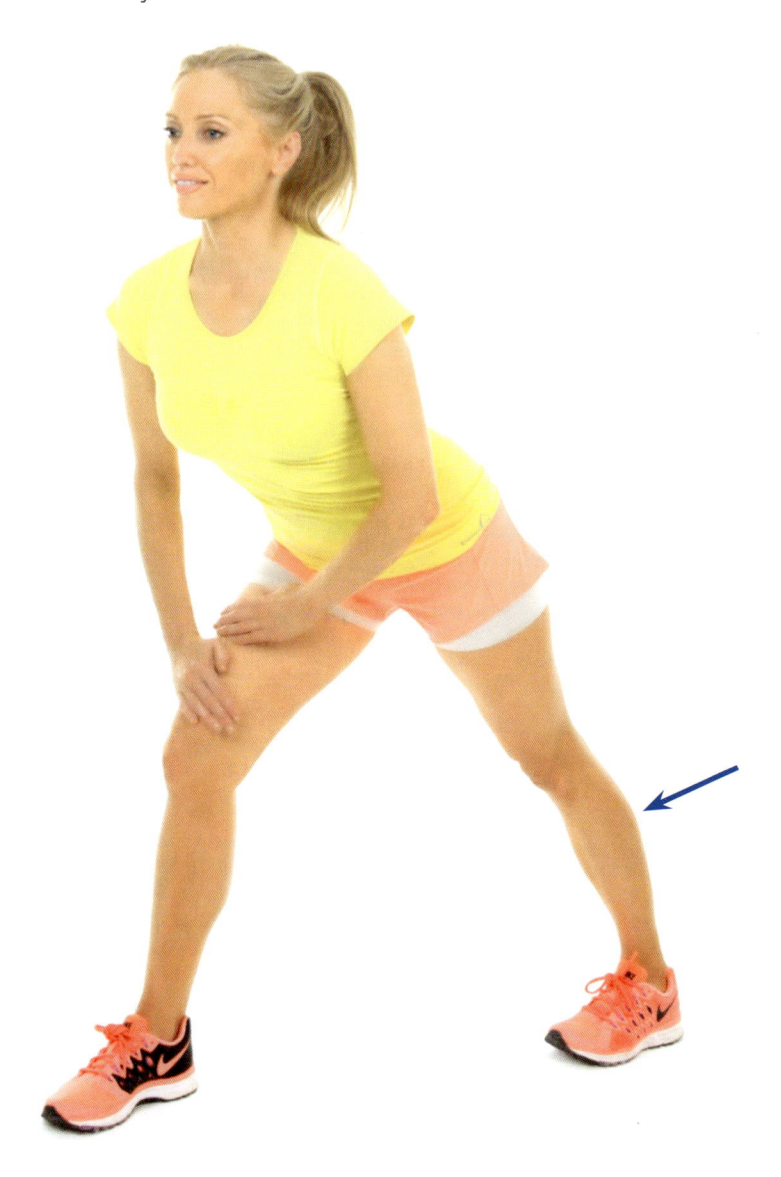

HAMSTRING STRETCH

Place one leg in front, heel on the floor, and bend the knee of the back leg. Then place both hands on the supporting leg and feel the stretch all the way through the back of the straight Leg. Hold for 10 seconds for your warm-up and 20 seconds for your cool-down.

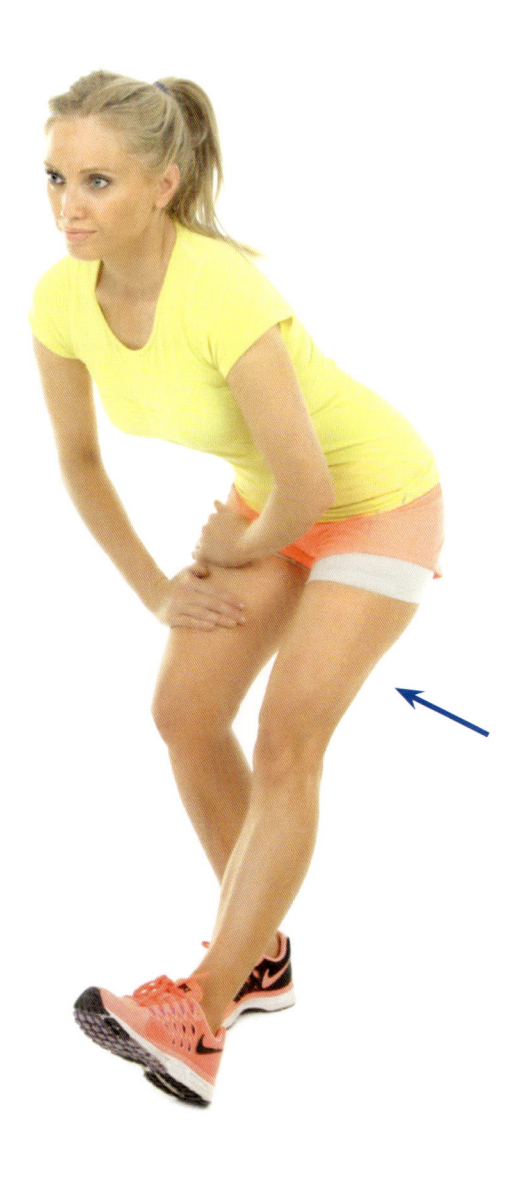

HIIT—HIGH-INTENSITY INTERVAL TRAINING

QUADRICEPS STRETCH

Stand with good posture and bend one leg behind you, bringing the foot toward the buttock. Gently hold the foot or sock of the bent leg. Keep the supporting knee slightly bent.

Hold for 10 seconds on each leg for your warm-up and for 15 seconds on each leg for your cool-down.

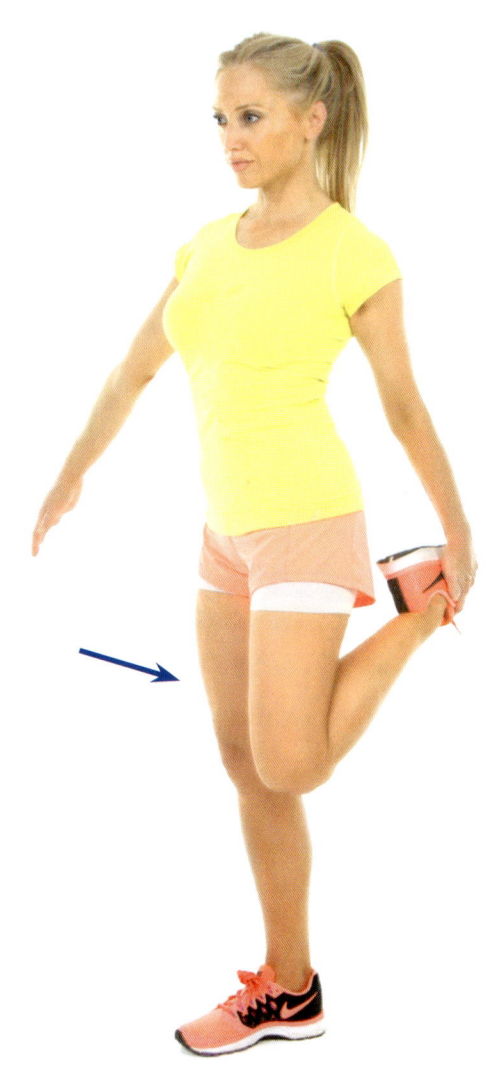

PART I | GETTING STARTED & UNDERSTANDING HIIT

TRICEPS STRETCH

Stand with a strong, firm, straight back, with knees slightly bent and tummy pulled in. Lift one arm up and bend it behind your head, aiming to get your hand between your shoulder blades. Gently support it with your other arm. For your warm-up, hold for 10 seconds then repeat with other arm. For your cool-down, hold for 15 seconds on each arm.

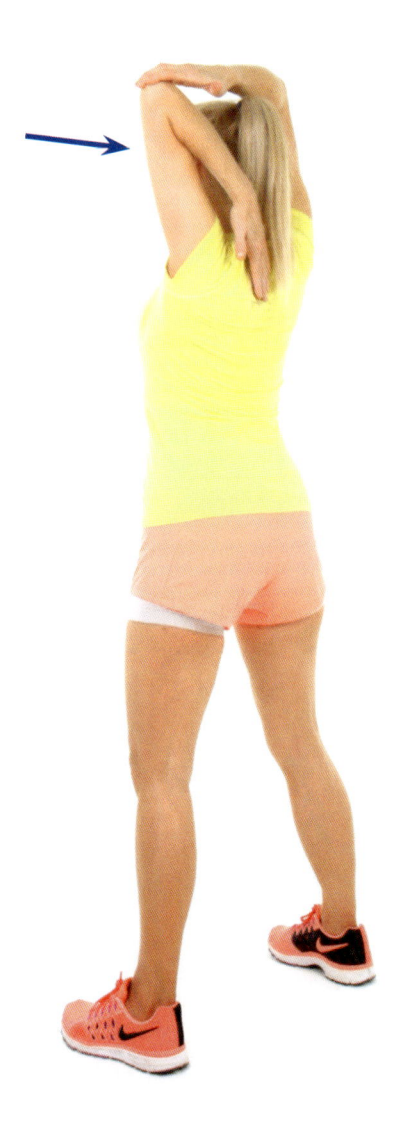

CHEST STRETCH

Stand with good posture and bring your arms behind you, lifting your shoulders up and back to feel the stretch in the chest. Hold for 10 seconds for your warm-up. Hold for 15 seconds for your cool-down.

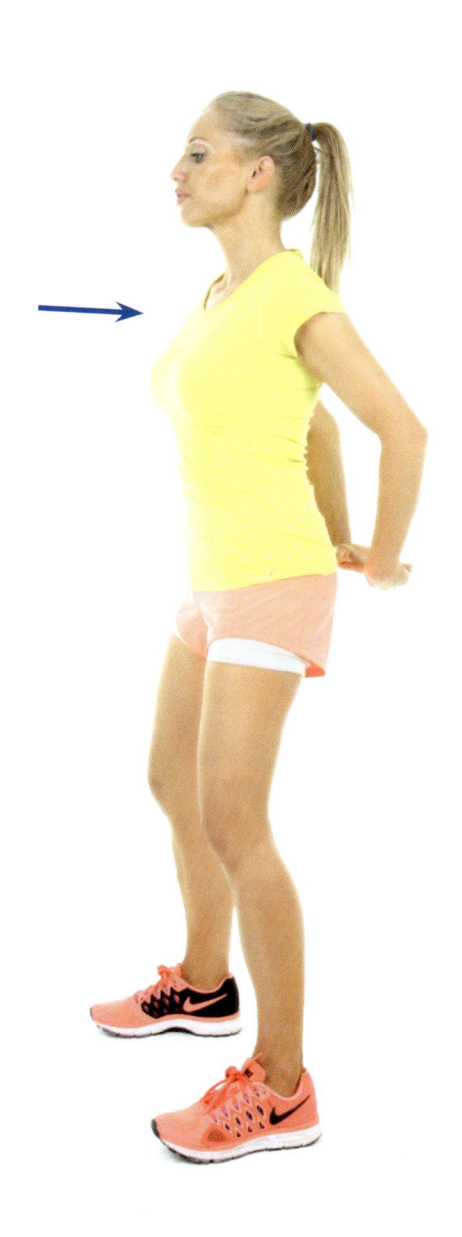

BACK STRETCH

Stand with good posture. Keep the knees soft and tummy pulled in. Hold your arms in front of you and imagine you are hugging a big beach ball, feeling the stretch in the back. Hold for 10 seconds for your warm-up. Hold for 15 seconds for your cool-down.

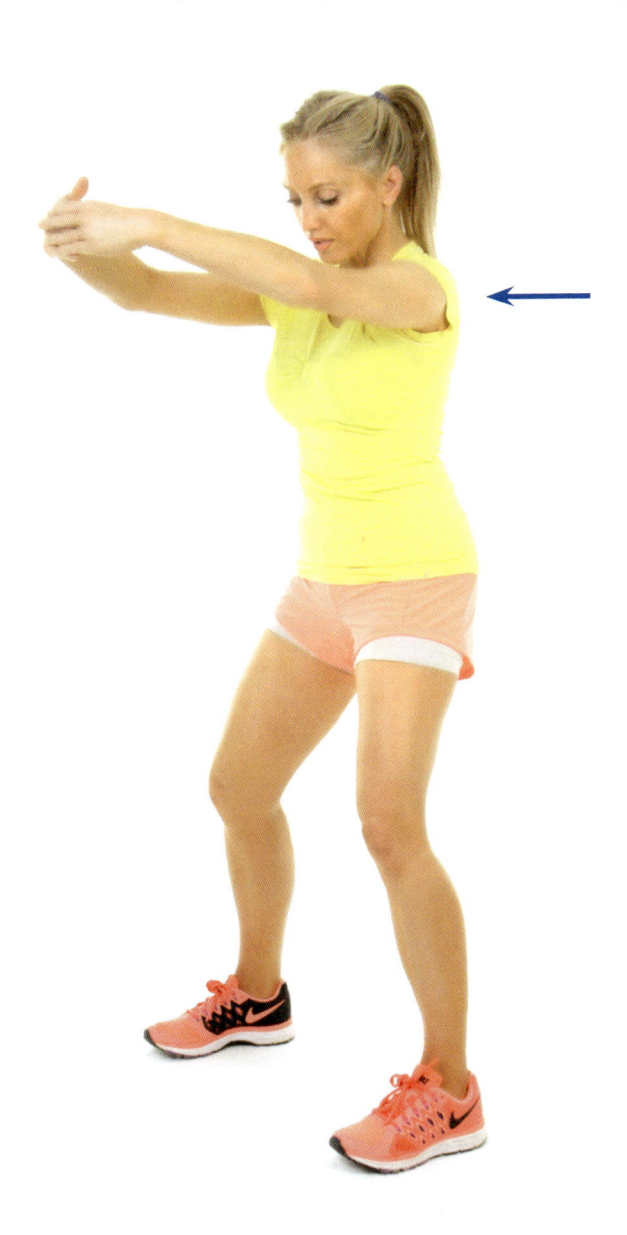

HIIT—HIGH-INTENSITY INTERVAL TRAINING

8 HEALTH AND SAFETY

This is one of the most important sections to read in this book, because your health and safety is the most important thing, and you should always apply these rules when you work out.

YOU SHOULD ALWAYS:

- Warm up, stretch, and then cool down as part of your workouts.
- Listen to your body, if something hurts or doesn't feel right, then stop.
- Drink plenty of water.
- If outdoors, then wear sunscreen and avoid the midday sun.
- If outdoors, always take a mobile phone with you and always let someone know where you are going.
- If outdoors, wear bright clothing.

AND NEVER:

- Work out if you are feeling unwell.
- Be impatient after an injury and rush back to exercise; be patient as it will pay dividends in the long run.
- Work out on an empty stomach.
- Exercise through pain.

AND MOST IMPOTANLTY, NEVER DOUBT YOURSELF AND ALWAYS FIND THE TIME TO DO ONE OF MY HIIT WORKOUTS.

9 IF YOU INJURE YOURSELF

The first thing you should do if you injure yourself when you are exercising is to stop immediately! It is recommended for any sprains, inflations, bruising, or swelling that you apply ice therapy straightaway to the place of injury.

Ice therapy is best applied to a fresh injury. When we injure ourselves, our blood flow increases to the injured area because this is the body's first step of healing itself. Such a rush of fluid actually compresses the nerves, which ultimately causes painful swelling. If the swelling isn't controlled, it can damage tissues further and therefore needs to be reduced. The benefits of applying ice will be to

- reduce bleeding into the tissues,
- prevent or reduce swelling (inflammation),
- reduce muscle pain and spasms, and
- reduce pain by numbing the area and by limiting the effects of swelling.

HIIT—HIGH-INTENSITY INTERVAL TRAINING

THERA°PEARL ICE PACKS are available at www.therapearl.com.

The effects of reducing swelling all help to prevent the area from becoming stiff by reducing excess tissue fluid that gathers as a result of injury and inflammation. Whether it's a torn ligament, bruising, or sore muscles, ice packs are easily popped into the freezer and then applied to protect your body from recurring pain and lasting damage. When I am training, I always take a THERA°PEARL ice pack with me just in case, and the great thing is that it molds to your body so you can apply compression to the injured area with ease. You should only ever apply ice therapy for 20 minutes, and never apply ice therapy

- to areas of skin with poor sensation to heat or cold,
- over areas of the body with known poor circulation,
- if you have diabetes, or
- in the presence of infection.

Make sure you allow a complete recovery from any injury before you rush back into exercise. As frustrating as it is to wait, you can simply end up making an injury worse, and it is always a good idea to get any injury checked out by a doctor or a specialist.

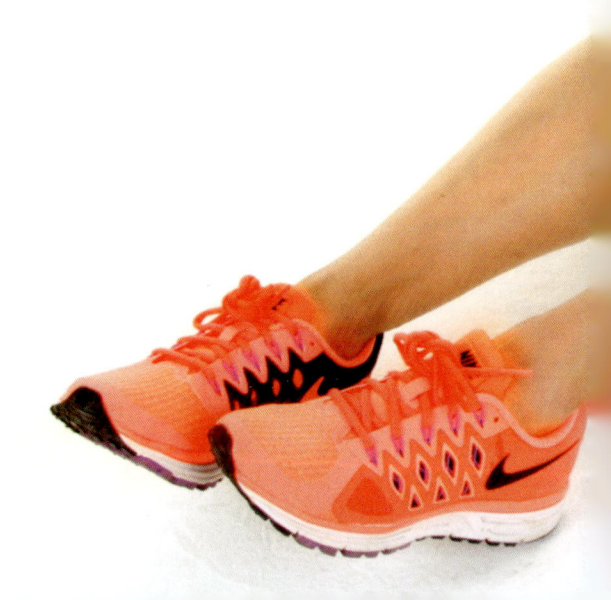

PART I | GETTING STARTED & UNDERSTANDING HIIT

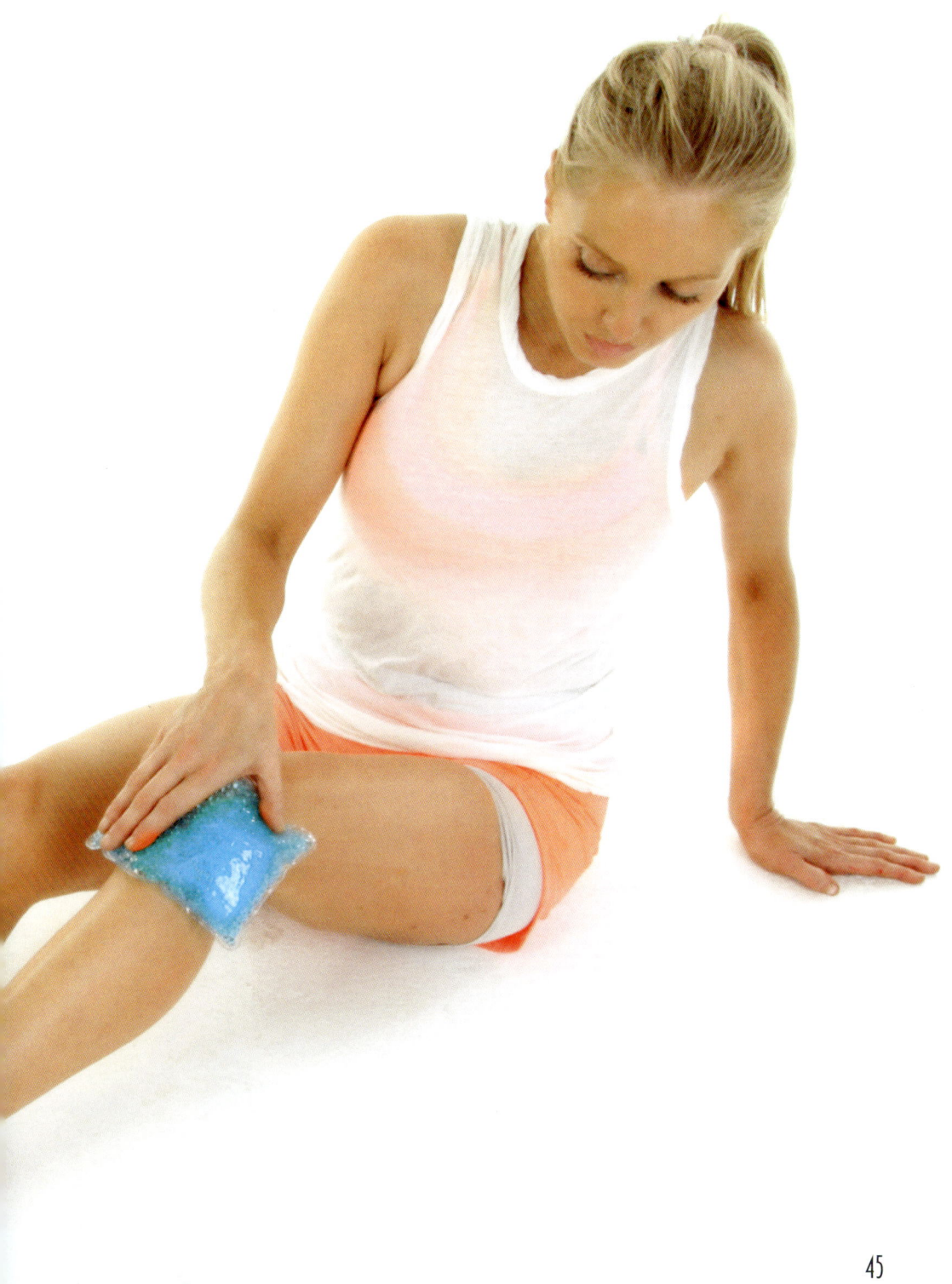

HIIT—HIGH-INTENSITY INTERVAL TRAINING

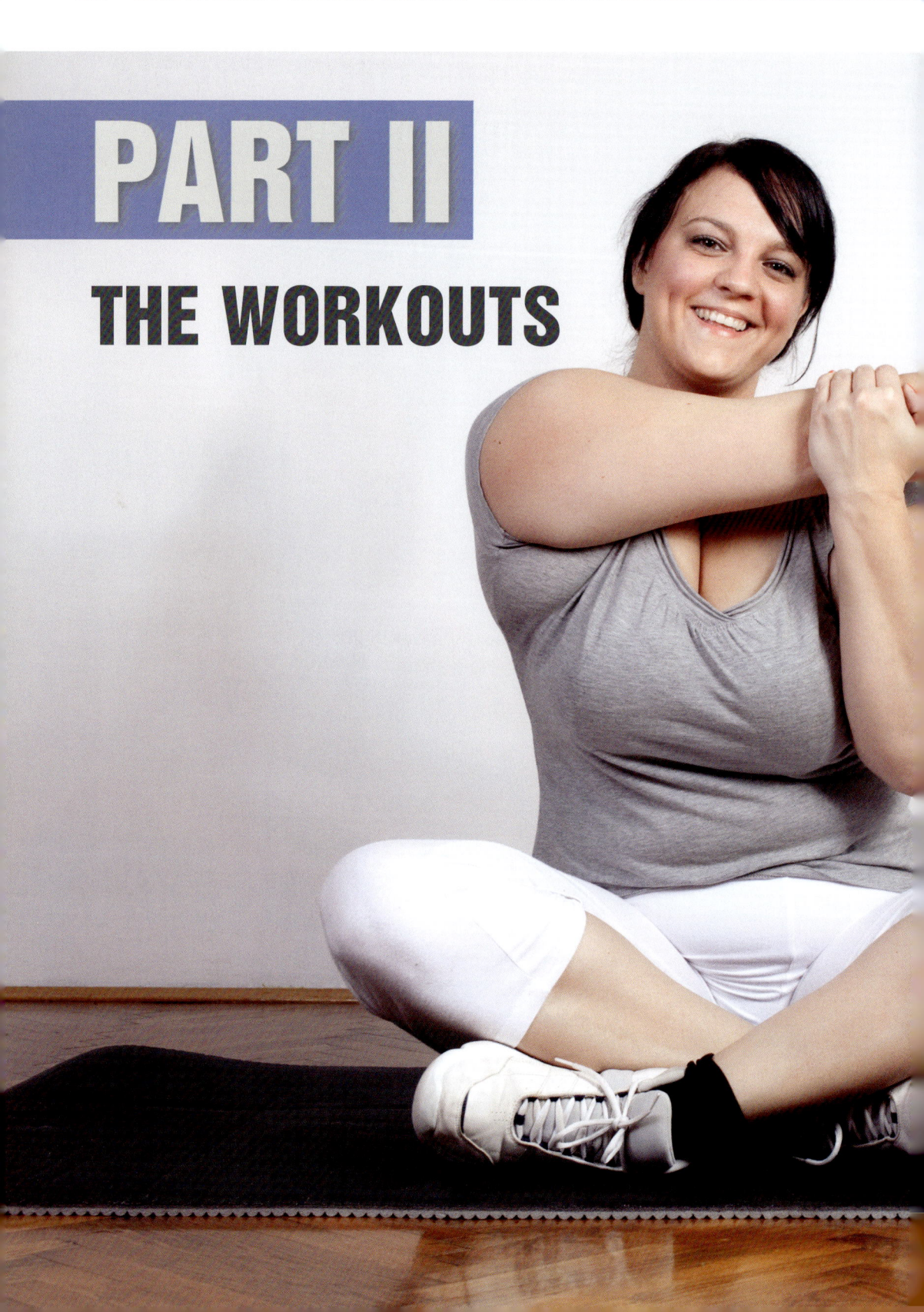

PART II
THE WORKOUTS

10 THE 4-MINUTE FAT-BURNER HIIT WORKOUT

- Time: 4 MINUTES
- Intensity: HARD
- Timed/Reps: TIMED
- Planes of Movement: SAGITTAL and FRONTAL
- Tones: THIGHS, BOTTOM, ABS, and ARMS
- RPE: 5 to 7

This one is short and sweet! And you will need a stopwatch for this. This workout has just two moves, which are the fat burners, plus a simple marching in place move, which is your rest exercise between the challenging exercises. They are both dynamic moves, and they engage multiple muscle groups and tone and sculpt you all over. As with all my workouts, this one will leave your body burning calories at a much higher rate for hours and hours after the workout. It is important to complete your warm-up and stretches, which can be found on pages 35-41.

HIIT—HIGH-INTENSITY INTERVAL TRAINING

EXERCISE 1: DEEP SQUAT STAR

Starting in a deep squat position, hold the squat and then jump up as high as you can, aiming to get your arms and legs out wide. Then land back into your deep squat position. Repeat this for exactly 20 seconds.

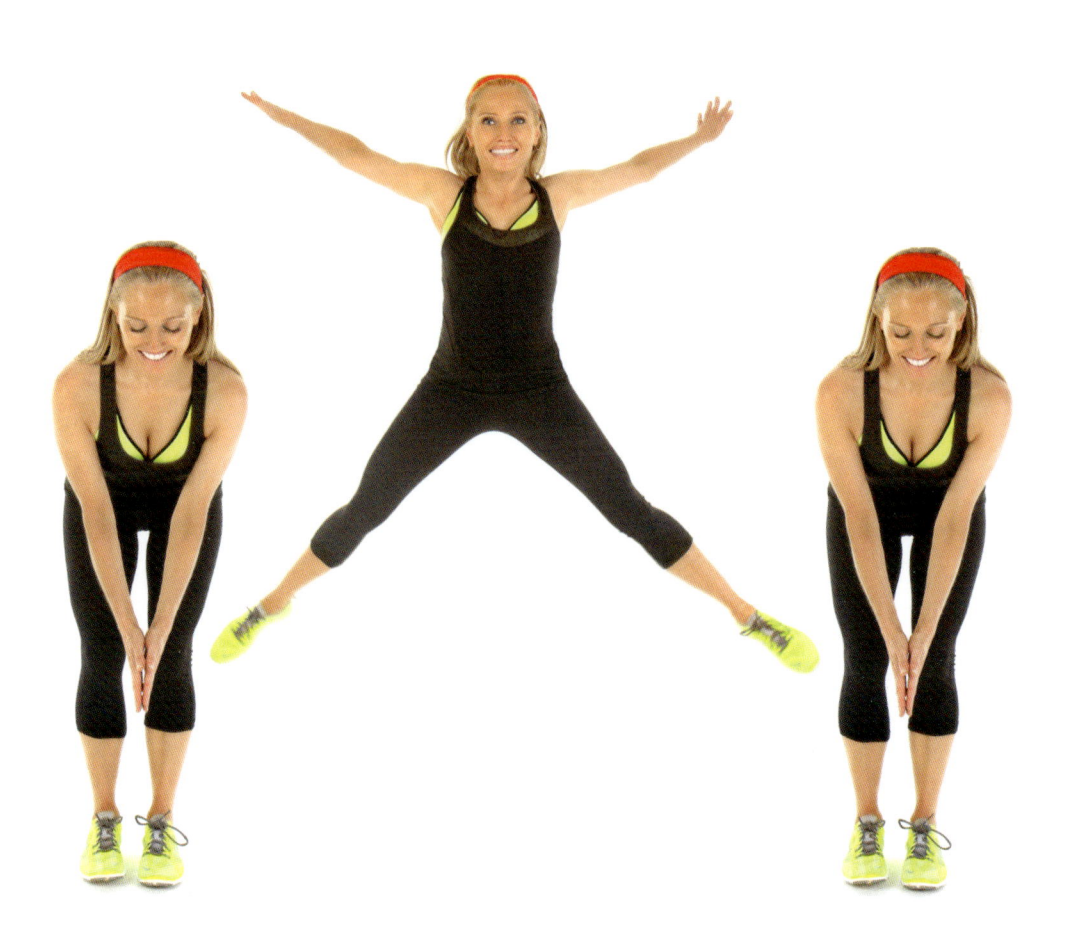

PART II | THE WORKOUTS

Then go straight into 10 seconds of marching in place. This is your recovery time, so you don't need to march fast, but just keep your body moving and take in some nice deep breaths.

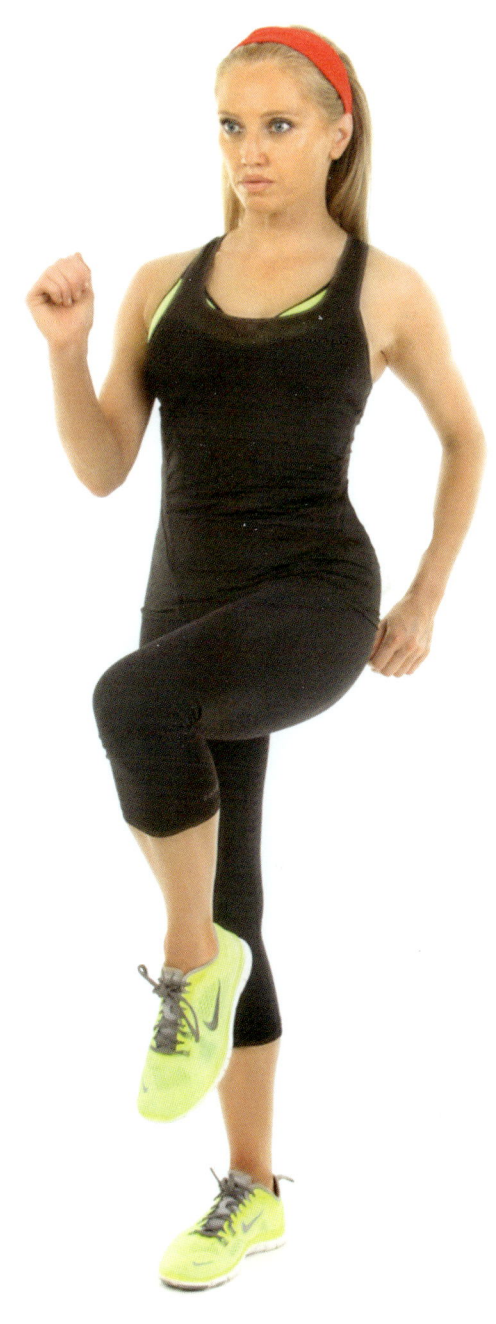

HIIT—HIGH-INTENSITY INTERVAL TRAINING

EXERCISE 2: MOUTAIN CLIMBER

After the 10 seconds of marching, go straight to the floor. With your hands slightly in front of your shoulders, bring one knee into the chest, hold, and then bring the other knee in. If you want a real challenge, then do this fast so it is just like you are running. Do this for exactly 20 seconds.

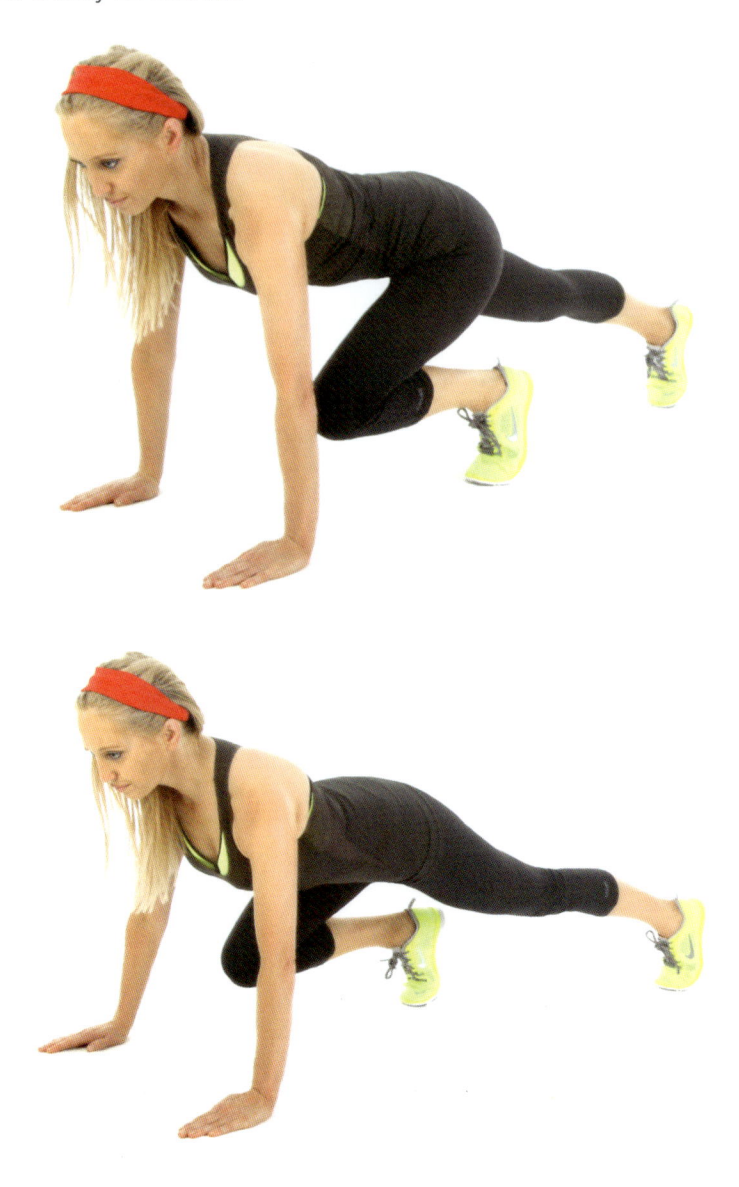

PART II | THE WORKOUTS

Then come straight back up to your march for exactly 10 seconds.

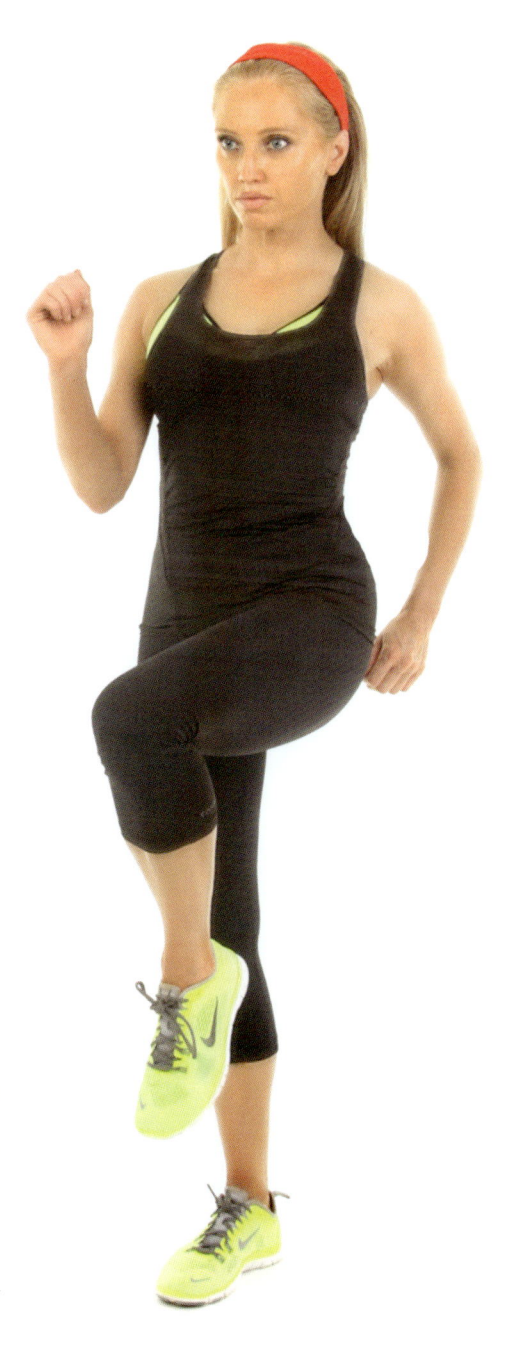

REPEAT THESE TWO EXERCISES NONSTOP another three times total, which will give an exactly 4-minute workout. Remember to do your cool-down stretches and drink a glass of water afterward.

HIIT—HIGH-INTENSITY INTERVAL TRAINING

11 THE 5-MINUTE HIIT WORKOUT

- Time: 5 MINUTES
- Intensity: MODERATE to HARD
- Reps: TIMED
- Planes of Movement: SAGITTAL, FRONTAL, and TRANSVERSE
- Tones: THIGHS, BOTTOM, ABS, ARMS, WAIST, and LEGS
- RPE: 5 to 7

Just 5 minutes is all you need. The exercises I have selected for this have a powerful mix of frontal moves which help to draw in your muscles from every angle. So the inches come off fast, and the high impact moves within this workout are great fast fat burners. Before you start, do your warm-up and stretches on pages 35-41.

PART II | THE WORKOUTS

EXERCISE 1: SKATER'S LUNGE

Keeping your hips square, place your right foot diagonally behind you, heel lifted. Lower into a lunge; don't let the front knee go past the toes. Extend the right arm across your body and the left out to the side. Now switch to the other side with a jump. (If you are a beginner to exercise, you can just step across.) Alternate from side to side for 50 seconds, with a 10-second rest period.

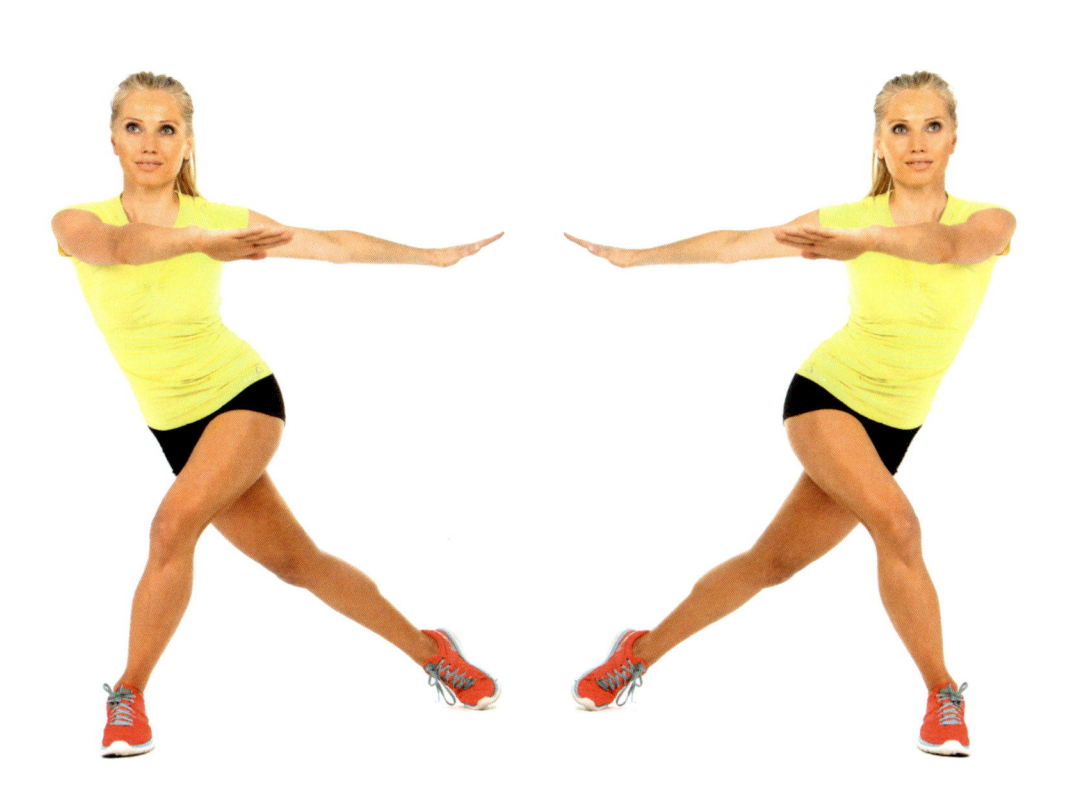

HIIT—HIGH-INTENSITY INTERVAL TRAINING

EXERCISE 2: ABDOMINAL ROPE PULL

Lying face up with your legs fully extended, imagine you have a piece of rope around your feet and use your hands to pull yourself up as high as you can. Cross one hand over the other, keeping your head and shoulders lifted. Repeat for 50 seconds, with a 10-second rest period.

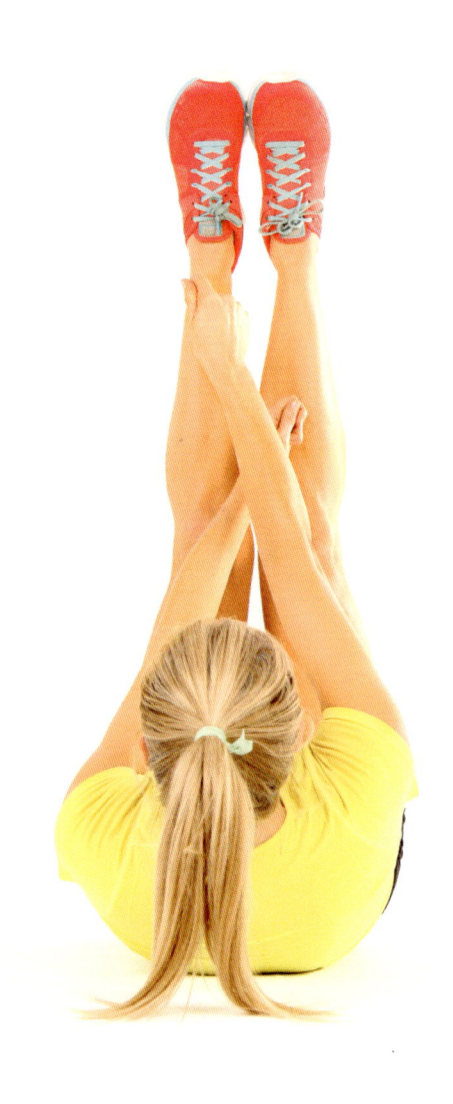

PART II | THE WORKOUTS

EXERCISE 3: CANNONBALL SQUAT

Start in a deep squat position and perform 3 deep squats, making sure you keep your knees behind your toes and sticking your bottom back. Then jump up high and land back in a deep squat. Squat 3 times and then jump again. Repeat for 50 seconds, with a 10-second rest period.

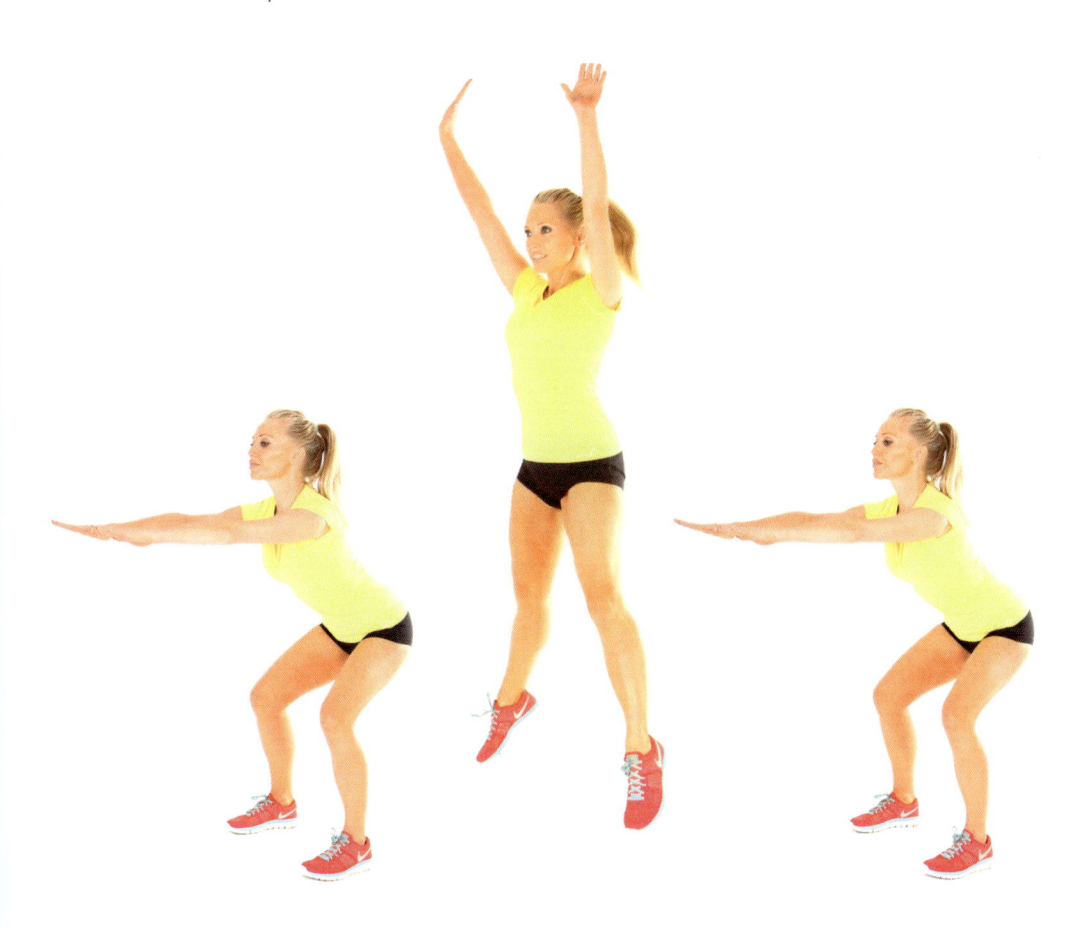

EXERCISE 4: PLANK LUNGE

Starting in a plank position, bring your right foot toward your right hand, hold, and then go back into a plank. Then bring the left foot to your left hand. Keep your tummy pulled in. Repeat for 50 seconds, with a 10-second rest period.

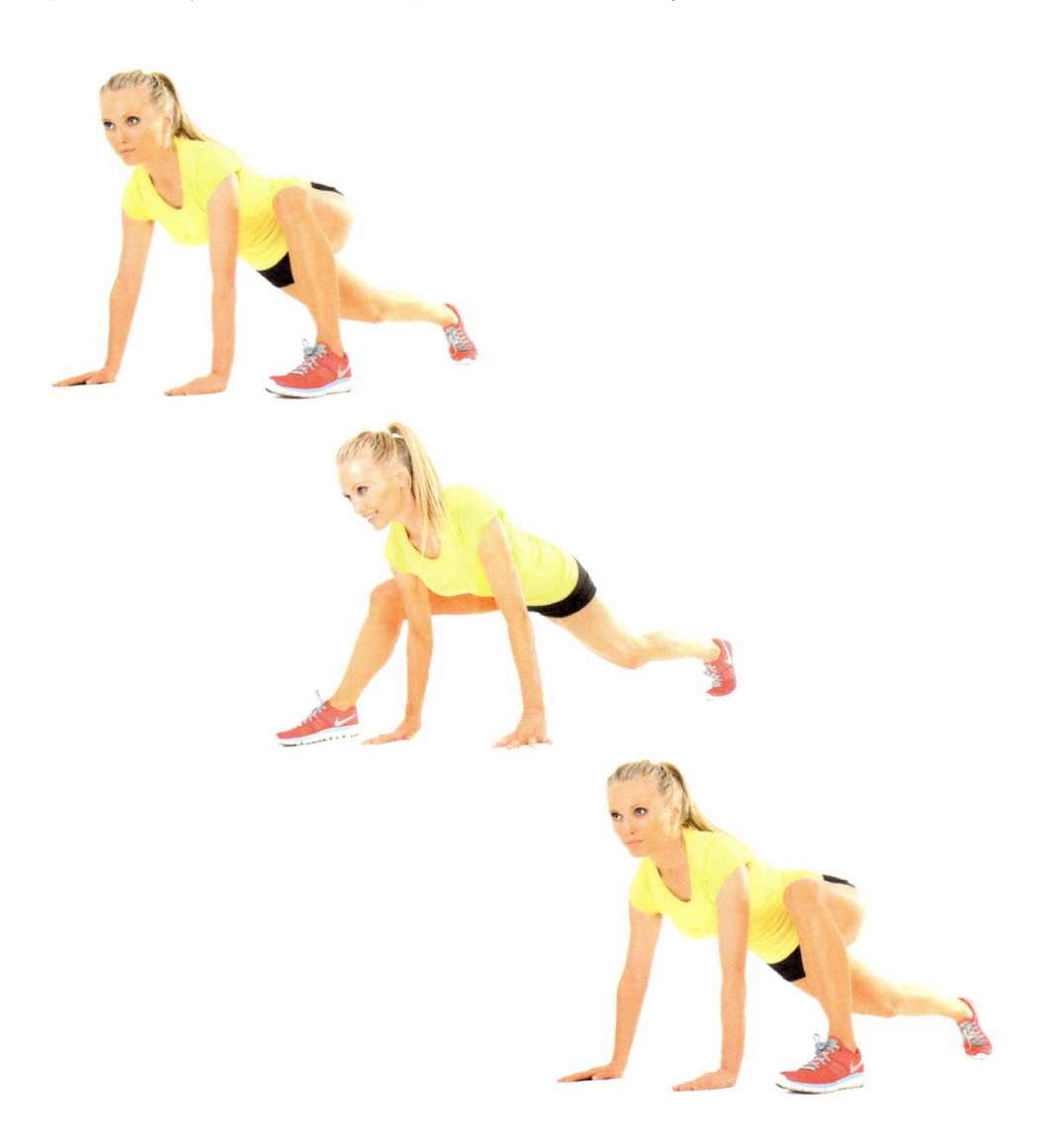

EXERCISE 5: WIPER WAIST MOVE

Start in a supine position with legs fully extended, keeping your knees over the line of your hips, toes pointing up, and your arms out to your sides, with your palms facing up. Now slowly lower to one side (only to a 45-degree angle), come back to center, and then lower to other side, constantly keep your tummy pulled in. Repeat for 50 seconds, with a 10-second rest period.

Complete your cool-down and stretches on pages 35-41. And drink a glass of water.

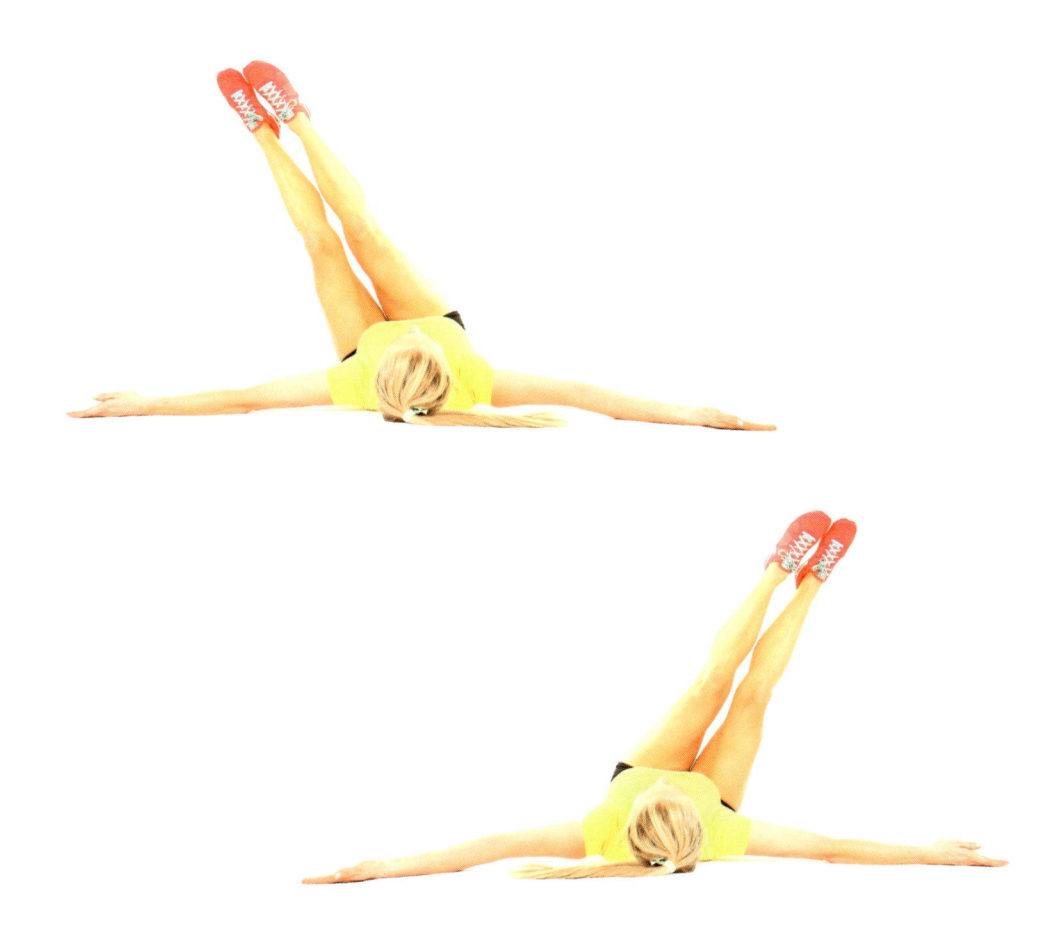

HIIT—HIGH-INTENSITY INTERVAL TRAINING

EXERCISE 2: LUNGE AND KICK

Start in a deep lunge position with your hands on your hips. Then kick your left leg straight out in front and lift your arms to shoulder height. Then return to the start position. Repeat for 25 seconds on the left leg and then do the same on the right leg. Follow with a 10-second rest period.

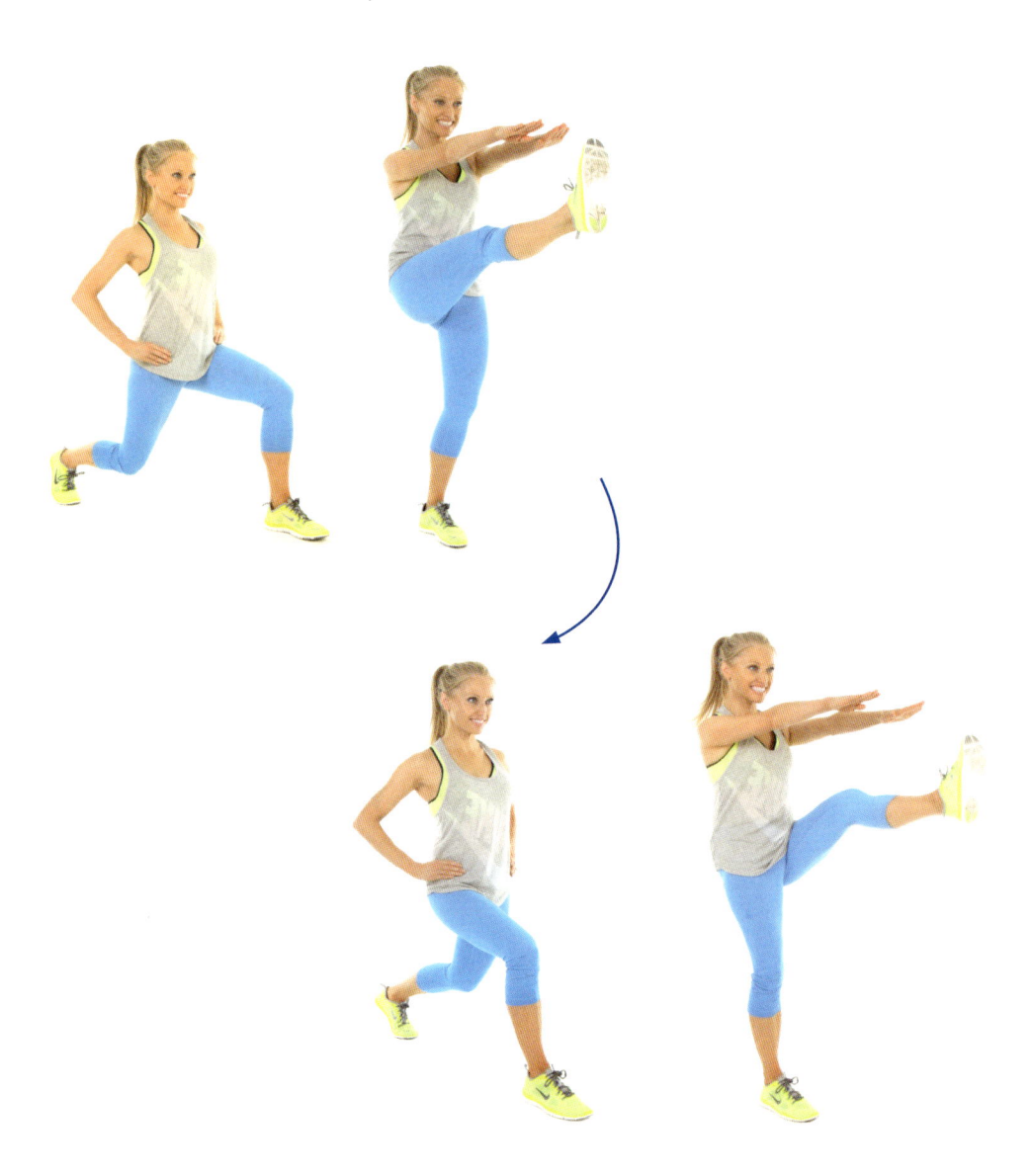

PART II | THE WORKOUTS

EXERCISE 3: JUMP UP

Start in a supine position with arms extendes above your head. Then come straight up to a standing position as fast as you can and jump high. Come straight back to the start position, and do this for 50 seconds. Then have a 10-second rest period.

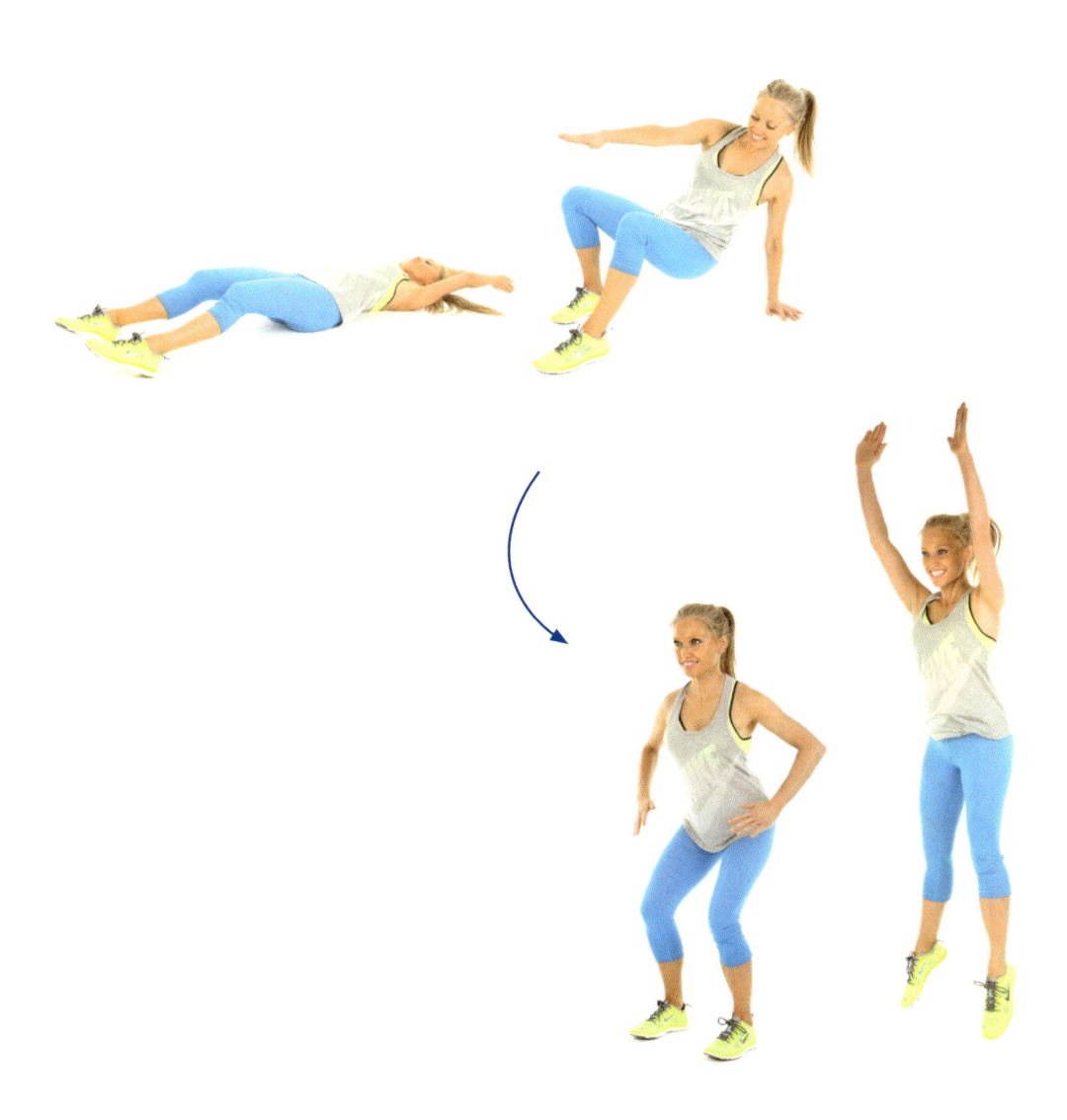

HIIT—HIGH-INTENSITY INTERVAL TRAINING

EXERCISE 6: AB SHAPER

Sitting on the floor with your knees bent and feet on the floor, rotate from your waist and reach your hands around to one side, hold, and then rotate to the opposite side. If you want to work those abs harder, then you can lean back slightly. Do this for 50 seconds, and then have a 10-second rest period.

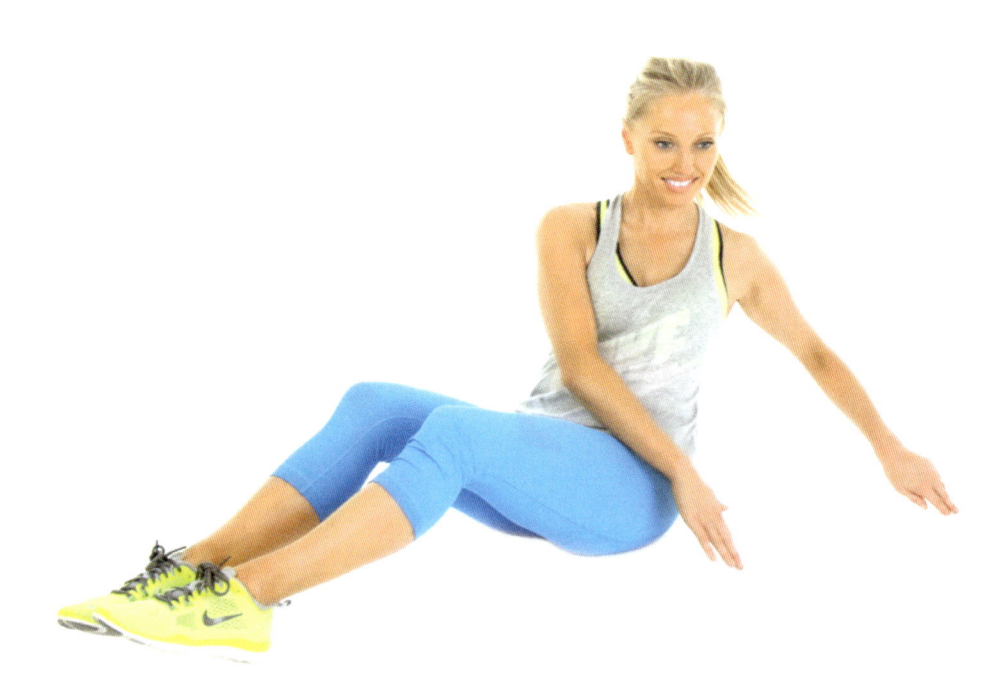

EXERCISE 7: FACEDOWN KNEE TO CHEST

On the floor with your hands slightly in front of your shoulders, bring one knee into the chest, hold, and then switch to the other knee. If you want a real challenge, then do this fast, so it is just like you are running. Do this for exactly 50 seconds, and then have a 10-second rest period.

At the end of the workout, you must complete your cool-down stretches on pages 35-41 and drink a glass of water.

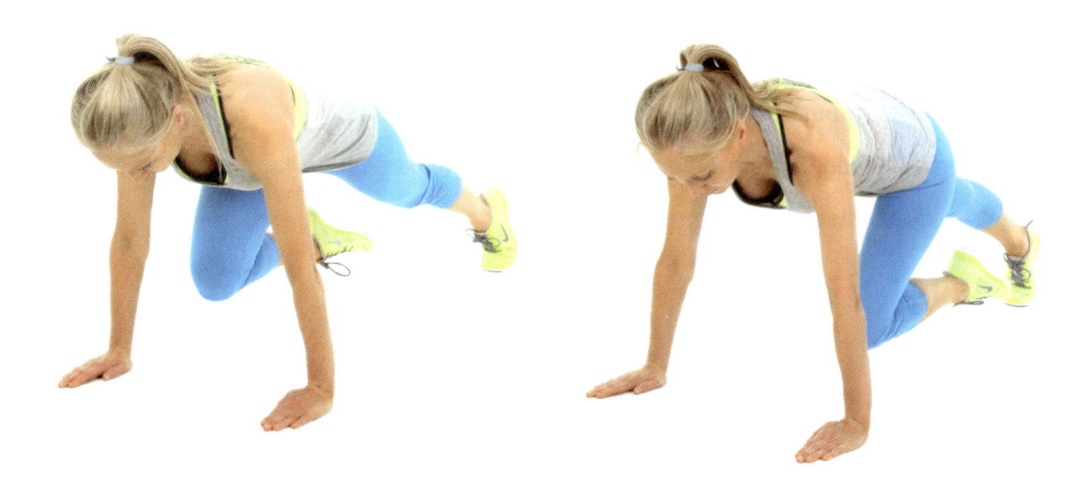

HIIT—HIGH-INTENSITY INTERVAL TRAINING

EXERCISE 2: KICK IT OUT MOVE

Start in a squat position. Make sure you squat low, but do not let your knees reach over the line of your toes. Extend your arms out in front and hold for a second. Then stand up and quickly kick one leg straight out in front while at the same time squeezing both your arms behind you, keeping your palms facing away. Come straight back to your squat position, hold, and then stand up and kick with the other leg. Keep doing this for 40 seconds, and then have a 20-second rest period in which you should just gently march in place.

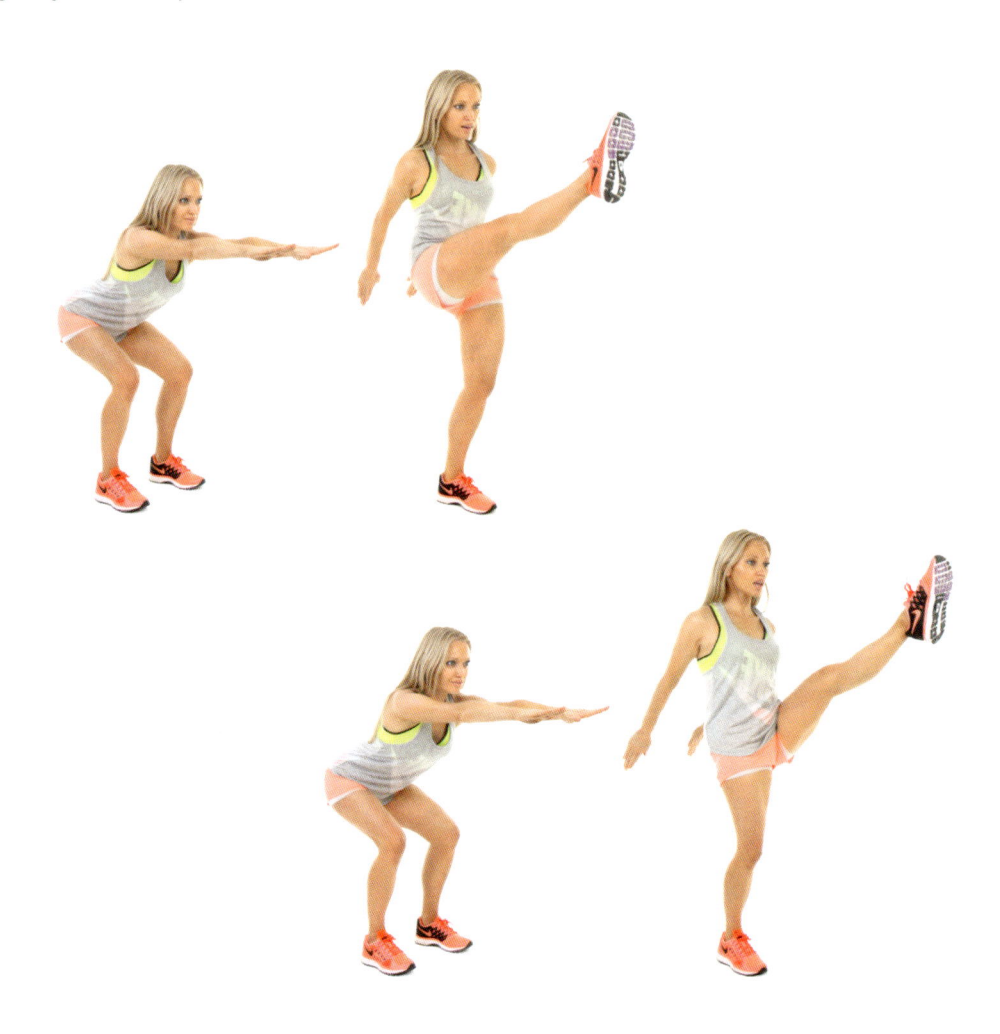

PART II | THE WORKOUTS

EXERCISE 3: 180-DEGREE TURN

Standing with good posture and tummy pulled in, face one side of the room. Now jump up and land so that you are now facing the opposite side of the room. The jump is the only high-impact move in this workout, so you can either do this as a very low and light jump or, if you want more of a challenge, as a high jump. Land softly, hold for a couple of seconds, and then jump back to the side of the room you faced at the start. Repeat for 40 seconds, and then have a 20-second rest period in which you should just gently march in place.

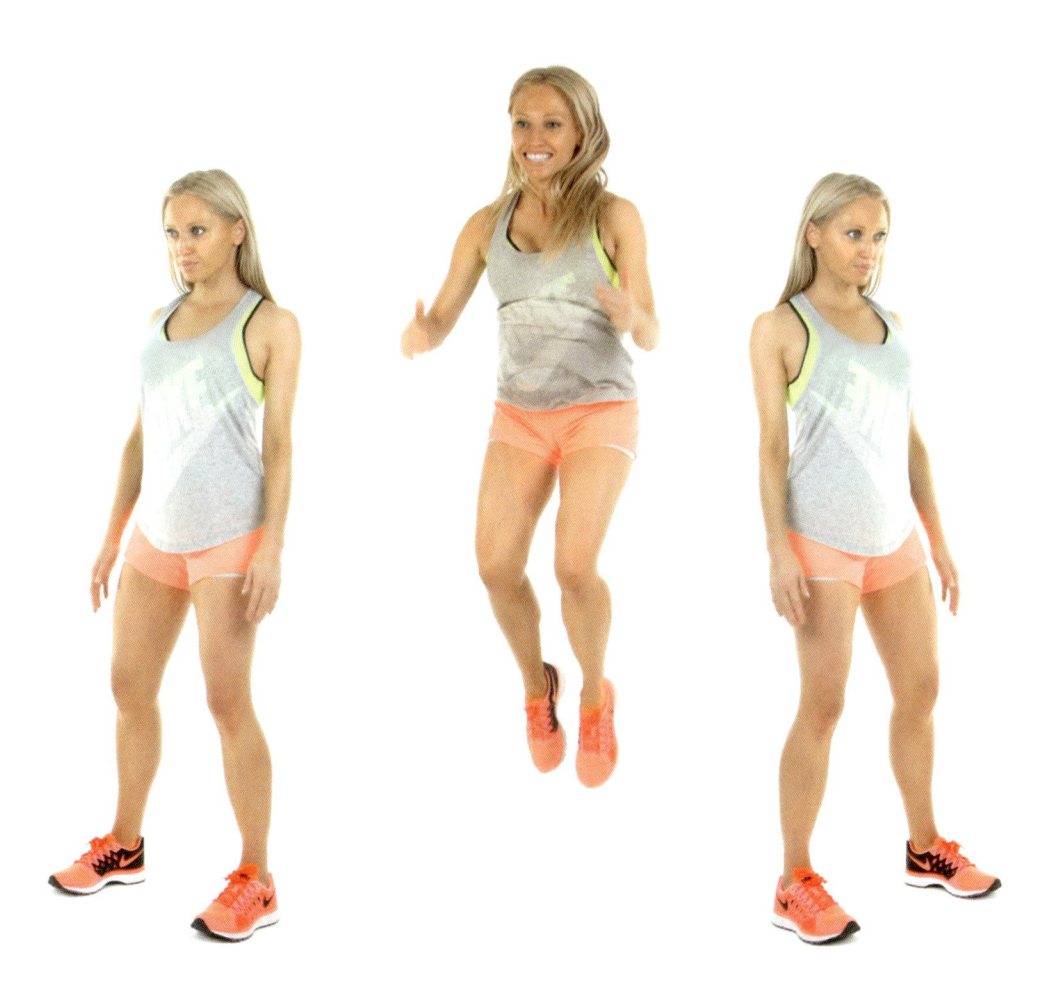

HIIT—HIGH-INTENSITY INTERVAL TRAINING

EXERCISE 1: BUNNY HOPS

Standing to the side of the bench, place hands firmly on the bench and have your knees slightly bent. Push off using your heels and your legs and jump over to the other side of the bench. Then immediately jump back to the other side. Do 40 repetitions, and then have a 10-second rest period.

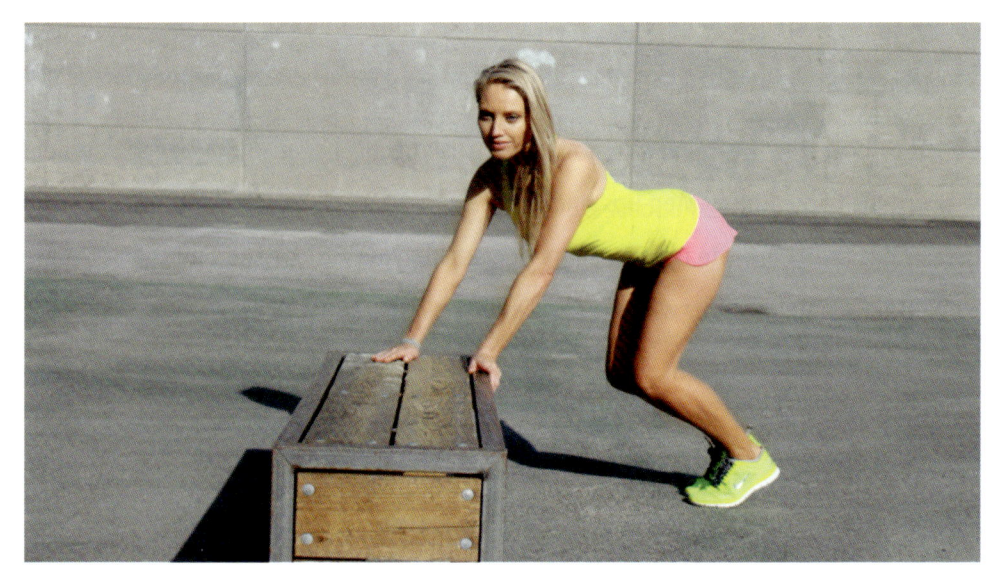

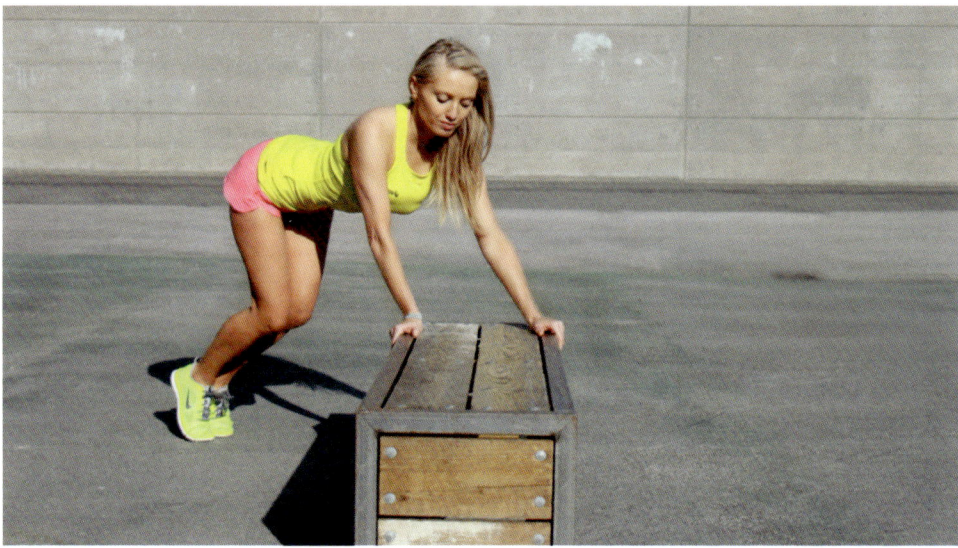

PART II | THE WORKOUTS

EXERCISE 2: BENCH PUSH-UP

Come into a push-up position, keeping the tummy pulled in tight. Your heels, hips, and head should all be in a straight line. As you perform the push-ups, be sure to constantly keep those tummy muscles pulled in. Do 25 repetitions (if you need to, you can do 15, then rest for 10 seconds, and then do the remainder).

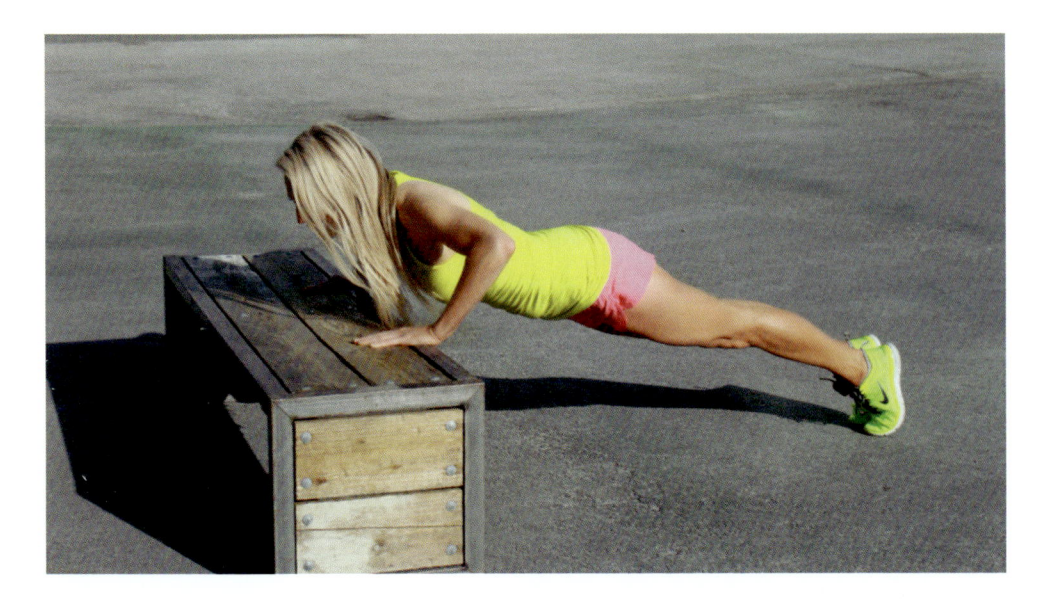

HIIT—HIGH-INTENSITY INTERVAL TRAINING

EXERCISE 3: STEP IT UP

Stand facing the bench and step up using the left leg. Do 20 step-ups on the left leg, and then switch legs and do 20 step-ups on the right leg. Maintain good posture throughout. If you want more of a challenge, you can add jumps.

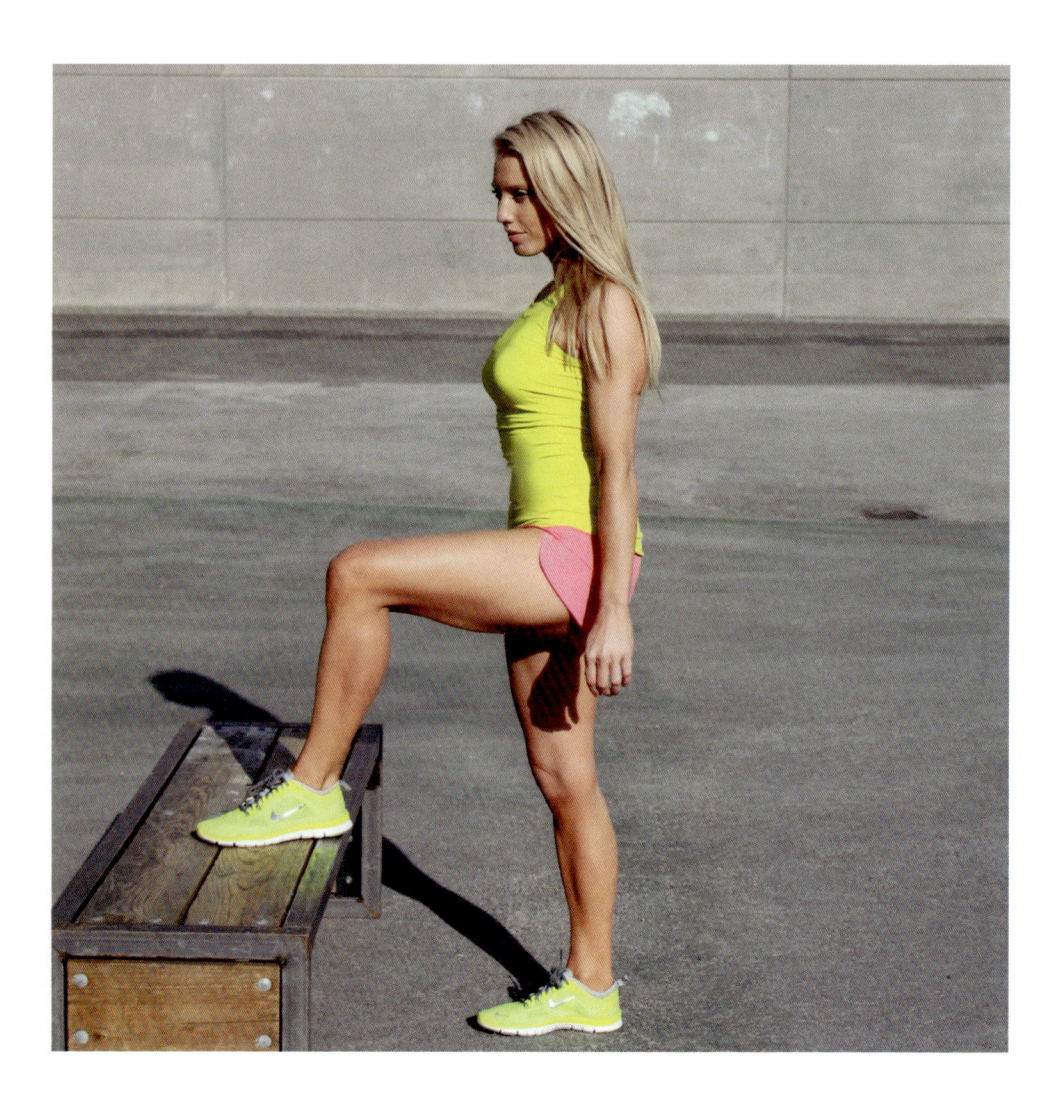

EXERCISE 4: ARM DIPS

Sit on the edge on the bench with your hands slightly wider than shoulder-width apart and your fingertips pointing forward, keeping your tummy pulled in. Lower your body down toward the ground by bending your elbows. Keep your shoulders pointing directly backward, hold for a second, and then push back up. Do 20 repetitions. If you want to make it harder, extend your feet farther out in front of you.

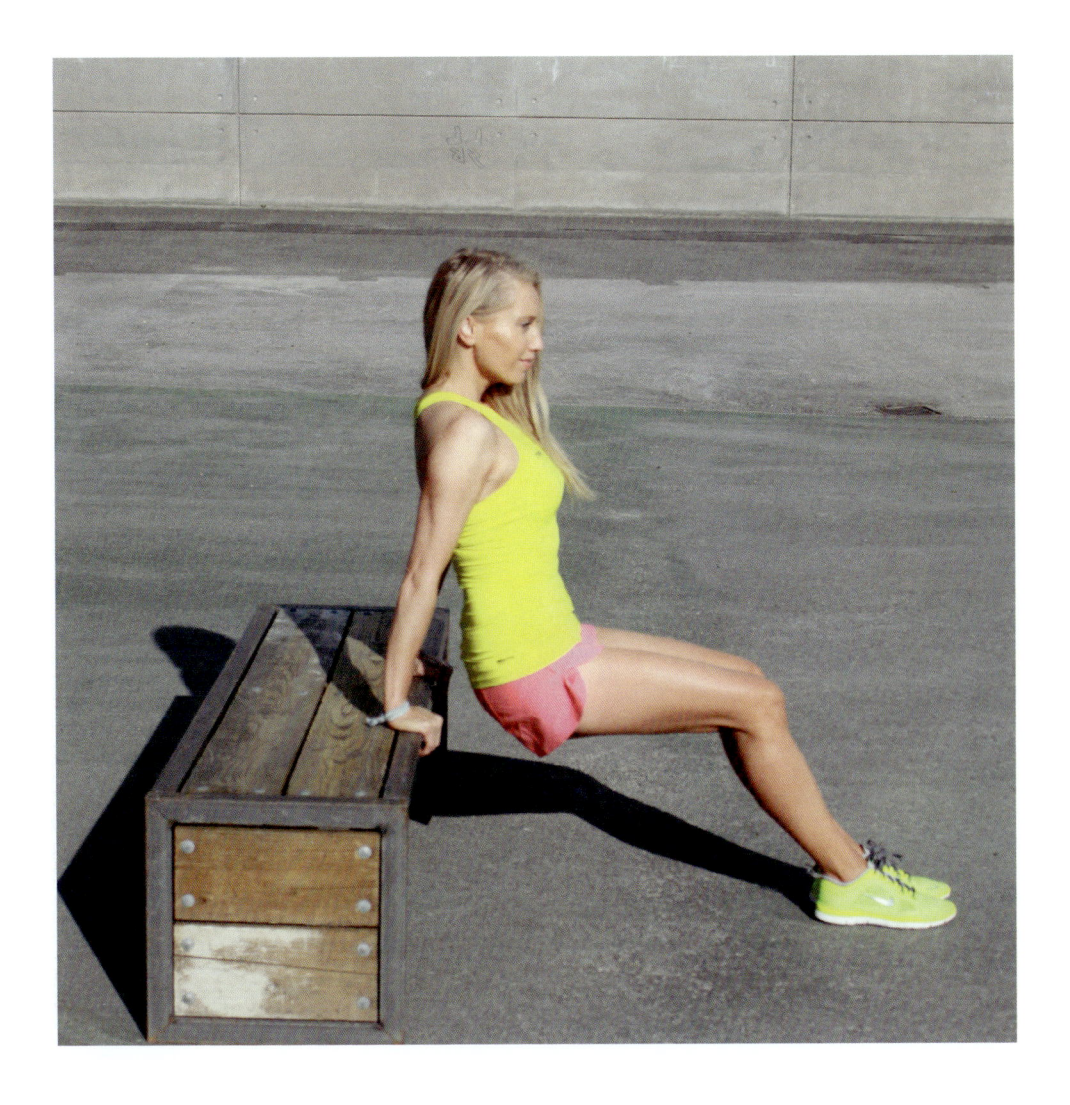

HIIT—HIGH-INTENSITY INTERVAL TRAINING

EXERCISE 5: STEP-UP KNEE LIFT

Start by standing by the side of the bench. Then step up with the leg closest to the bench, bring the opposite knee and arm up. Hold for a second and then lower back to start position. Do 20 repetitions on one side and then turn around to repeat on the other side.

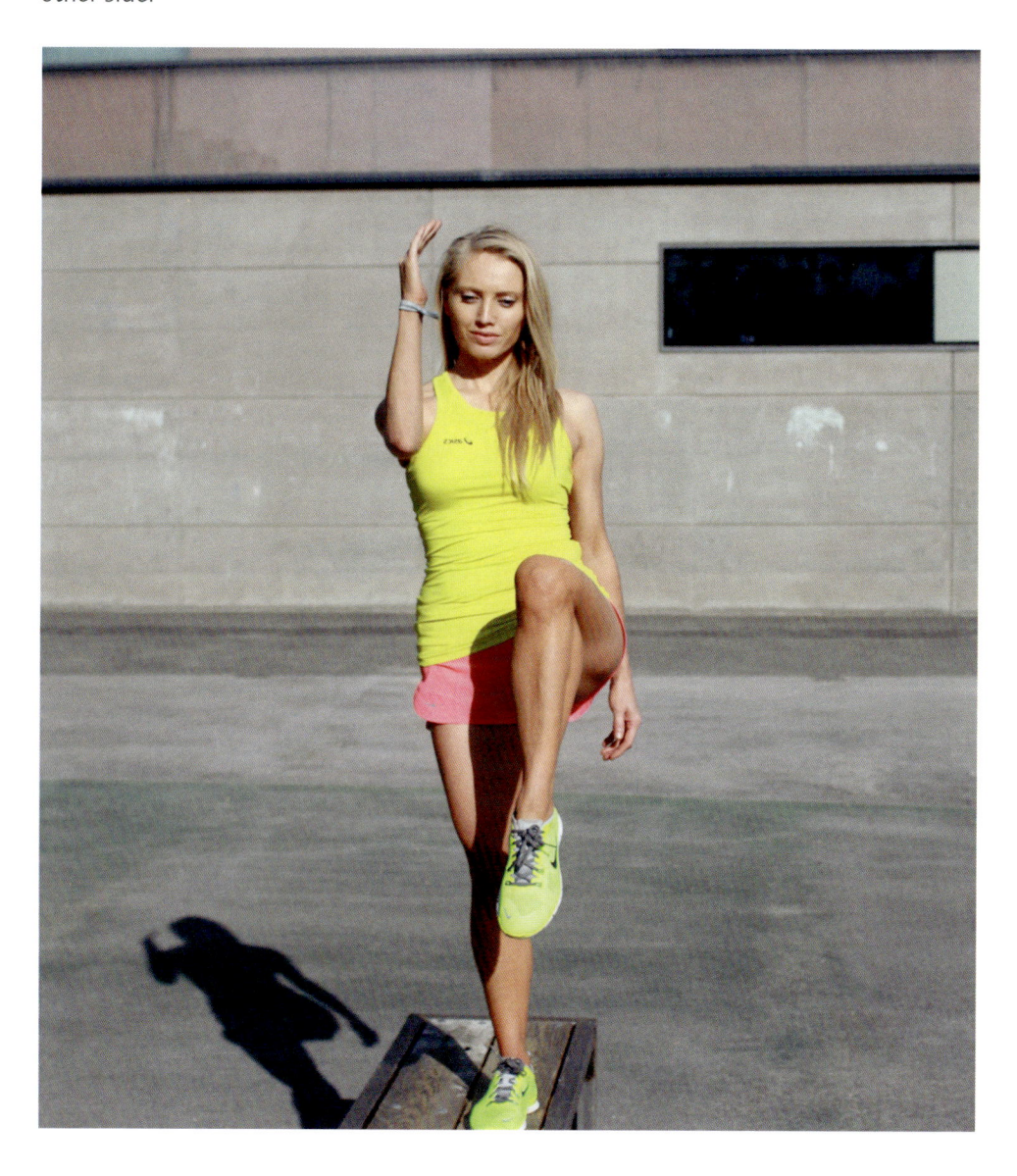

PART II | THE WORKOUTS

EXERCISE 6: V-CRUNCH

Sitting on the bench place, your hands behind you, firmly gripping the back of the bench. Lean back slightly and pull in your tummy muscles. Bend your legs and then slowly and controlled extend your legs away from your body and lean back a little farther as you bend the elbows. Hold for a second and then come back up to start position. Do 20 repetitions of these.

Take a 40-second rest period doing a gentle walk, and then repeat the whole routine again. Once completed, have a glass of water and perform all your cool-down stretches on pages 35-41.

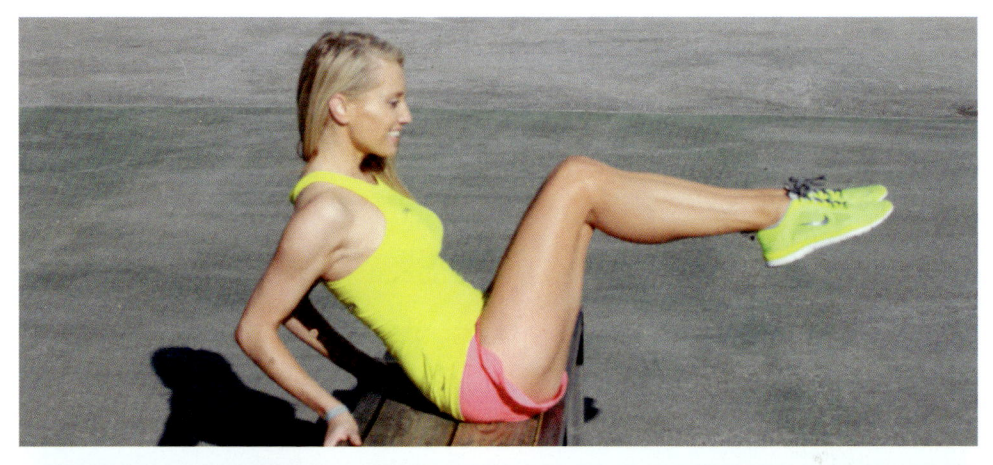

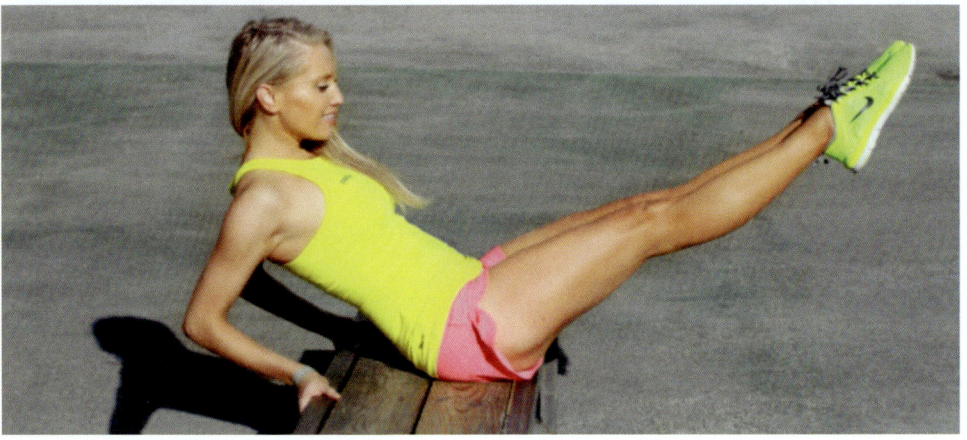

15 HOME HIIT CIRCUITS

- Time: Under 12 MINUTES
- Intensity: MODERATE to HARD
- Timed/Reps: REPS
- Planes of Movement: SAGITTAL, FRONTAL, and TRANSVERSE
- Tones: ABS, LEGS, BOTTOM, THIGHS, and ARMS
- RPE: 5 to 7

This workout can be done at home using the smallest amount of space, and you don't need any equipment (as with most of my workouts). Each move uses your own body weight as resistance, but you still get the full effects of toning, sculpting, and fat burning. Make sure you complete your warm-up and stretches on pages 35-41.

PART II | THE WORKOUTS

EXERCISE 1: T LUNGE

Start in a lunge position with your arms fully extended out to your sides and your palms face down and in line with your shoulders. Now push back up to a standing position, keeping arms out and upper body straight. Hold and then lunge back down with the opposite leg. Repeat this and do 50 repetitions. Then take a 10-second rest by marching in place.

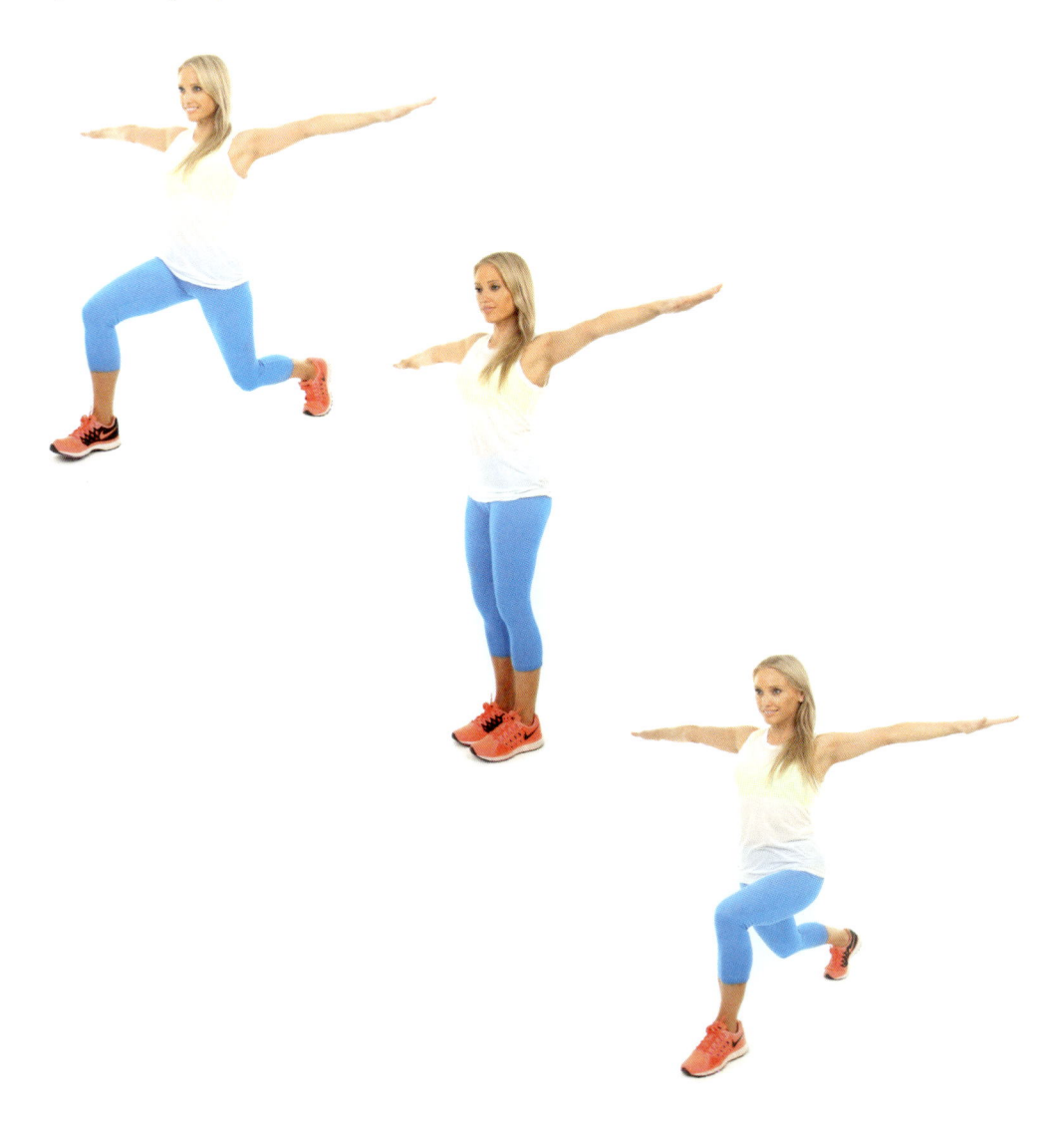

HIIT—HIGH-INTENSITY INTERVAL TRAINING

EXERCISE 2: SIDE DROPS

Start in a standing position with good posture and your arms fully extended in front of you at shoulder height. Now laterally lunge your left leg out to the side and touch the ground with your right hand. Hold for a second, and then push back up to the start position. Now this time lunge laterally with your right leg and touch the ground with your left hand. Repeat this exercise for 50 repetitions and then take a 10-second rest by marching in place.

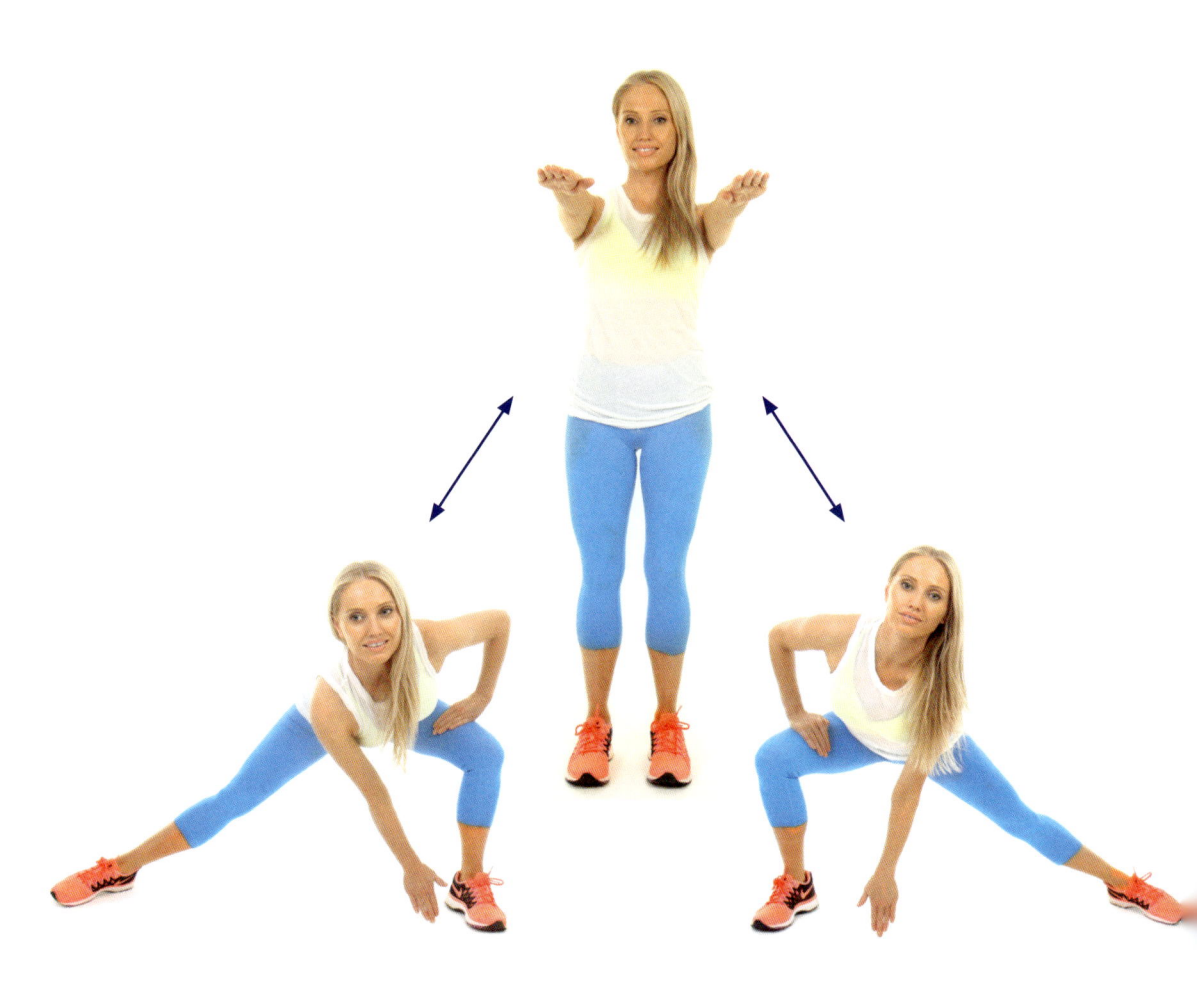

EXERCISE 3: PLANK LEG CROSS

Start in a fully extended plank position, keeping your belly muscles tight. With control, cross your left leg under to the right side, hold, and then come back into the plank position. Hold and then cross your right leg under to the left side. Keep alternating for 40 repetitions (or fewer if 40 is too challenging), and then march in place for a 10-second rest. Remember to keep those tummy muscles pulled in to protect your back.

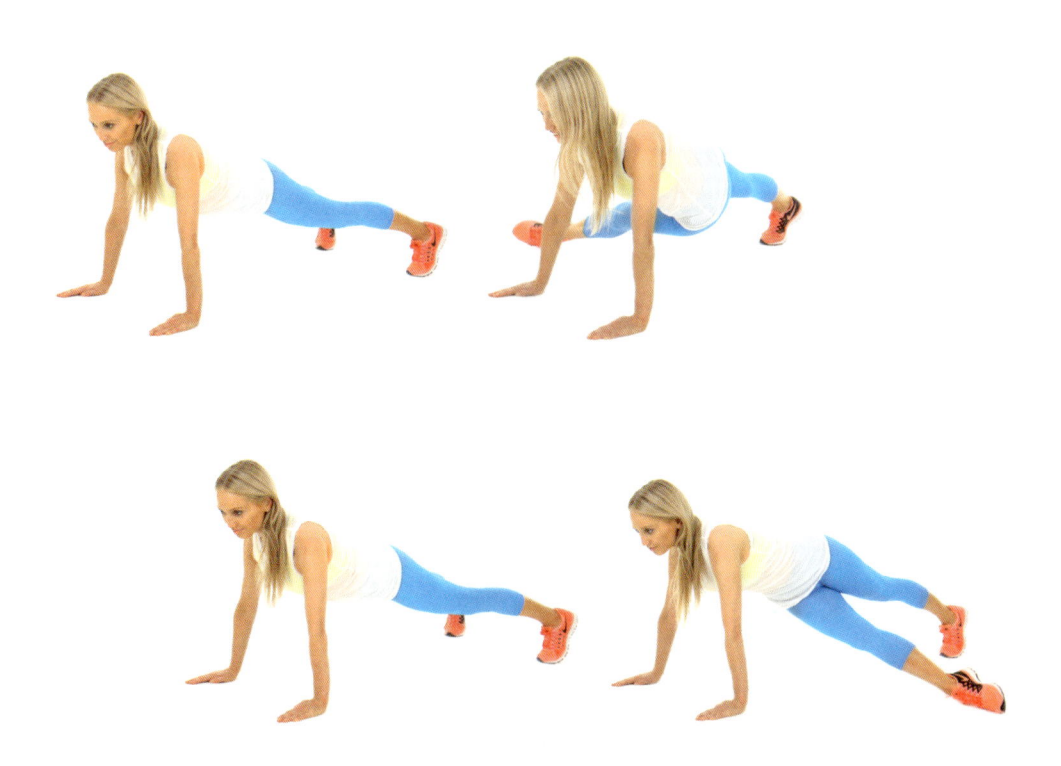

HIIT—HIGH-INTENSITY INTERVAL TRAINING

EXERCISE 6: HIGH AND LOW MOVE

Start on your tiptoes with your arms above your head. Come into a deep squat and try to touch the floor with your right hand. Hold for a second and then come straight back up onto your tiptoes with arms above your head. Lower into a deep squat again and try to touch the floor with your right hand. Repeat for a total of 40 repetitions and then march in place for a 10-second rest.

Once you have completed this round, have a drink of water, and then repeat it, but this time just perform 20 repetitions for each exercise. Then grab some more water and finally finish the last round by doing just 10 repetitions of each exercise. Then complete all your cool-down stretches.

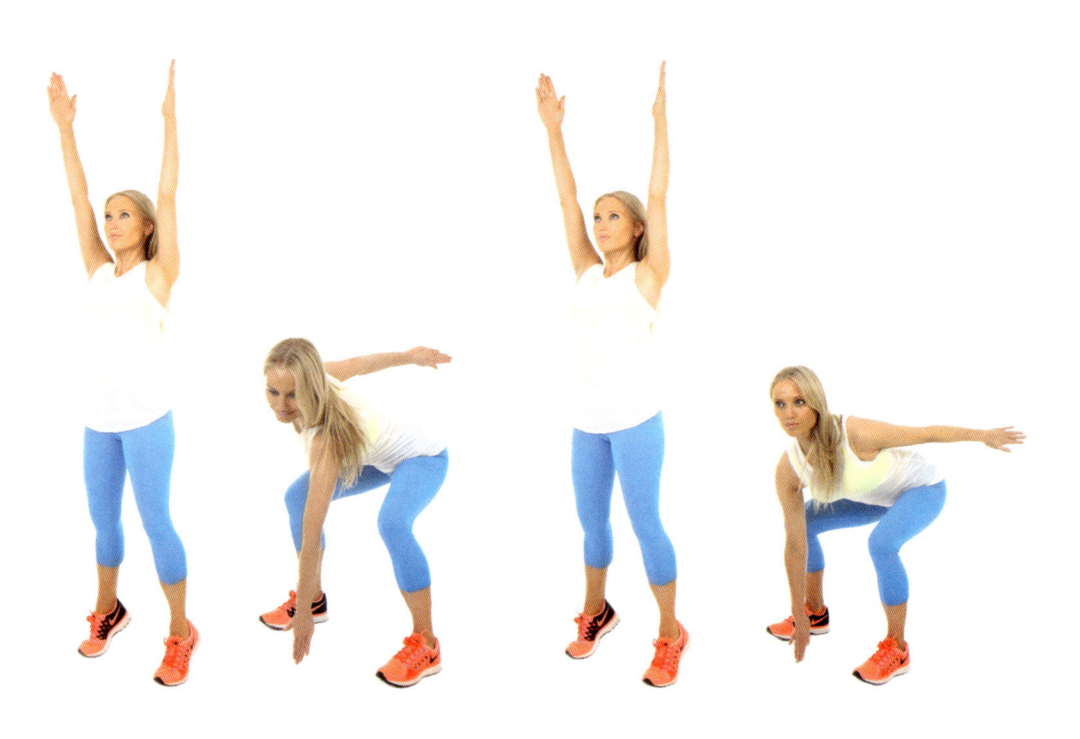

PART II | THE WORKOUTS

16 THE GET STRONG HIIT WORKOUT

- Time: Under 10 MINUTES
- Intensity: HARD
- Timed/Reps: TIMED and REPS
- Planes of Movement: SAGITTAL and FRONTAL
- Tones: BICEPS, SHOULDERS, BACK, CHEST, LEGS, ABS, BOTTOM, and CLAVES
- RPE: 5.5 to 7.5

This workout is all about building upper-body strength and increasing stamina and speed. The push-ups help to develop the arms, chest, and abs, and the plyometric jumps help increase stamina, speed, and endurance.

Before you perform this workout, complete your warm-up and stretches on pages 35-41.

HIIT—HIGH-INTENSITY INTERVAL TRAINING

EXERCISE 1: POWER SIDE-TO-SIDE SQUAT

Start in a deep squat position with arms in front of you. Jump up high to the right and land in a deep squat. Hold and then jump up high to the left, landing again in a deep squat. Do this for 40 seconds and then rest for 10 seconds.

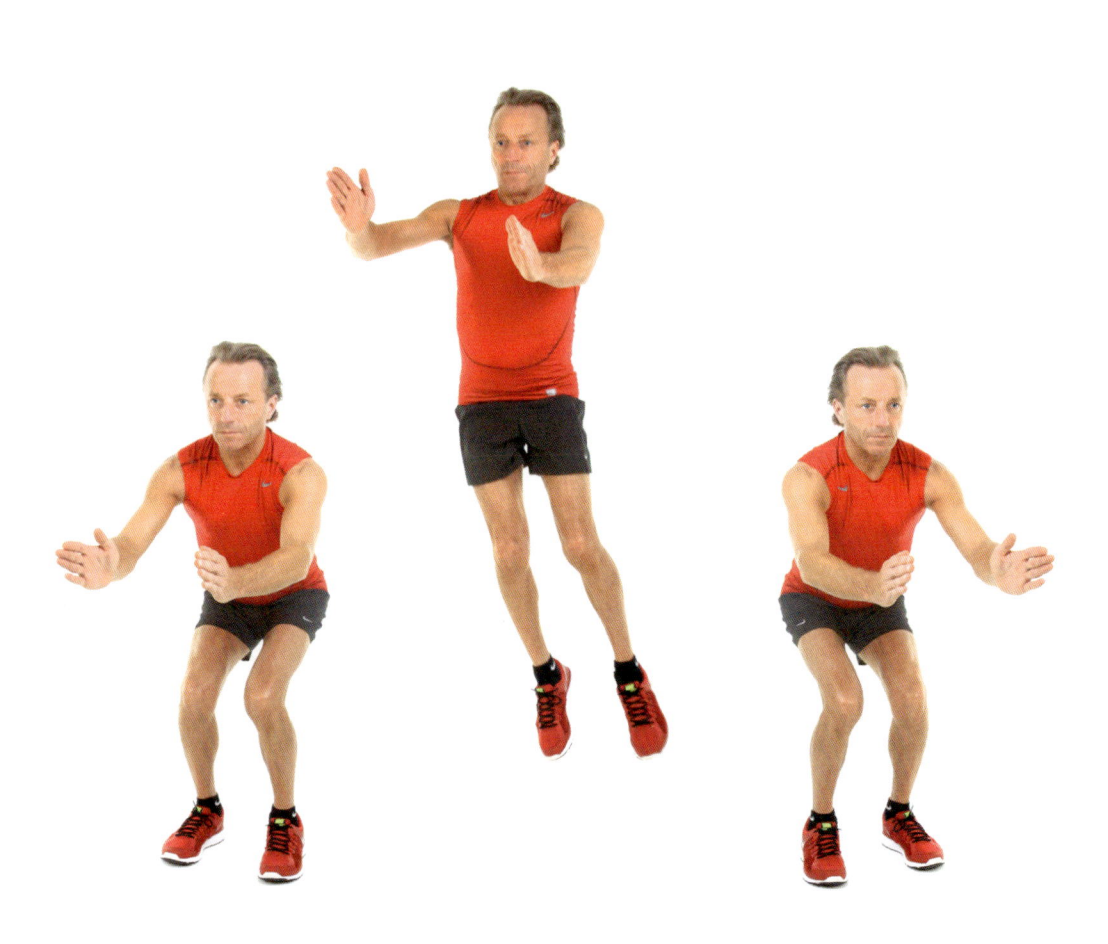

EXERCISE 2: PUSH-UP

Starting in a full push-up position, slowly lower your chest to the ground, keeping tummy muscles pulled in. Aim for 50 repetitions. If you need to rest, that's fine. Rest for 10 seconds. Come into a kneeling position to give the upper body a little rest. Then finish the remaining repetitions.

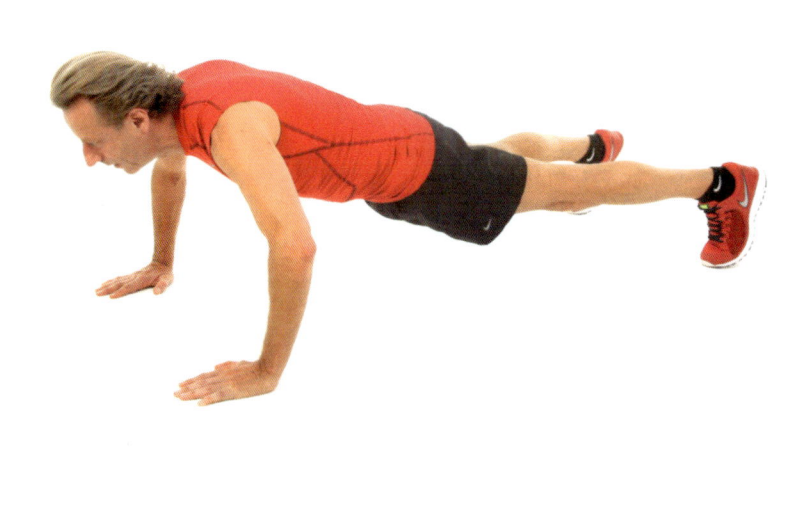

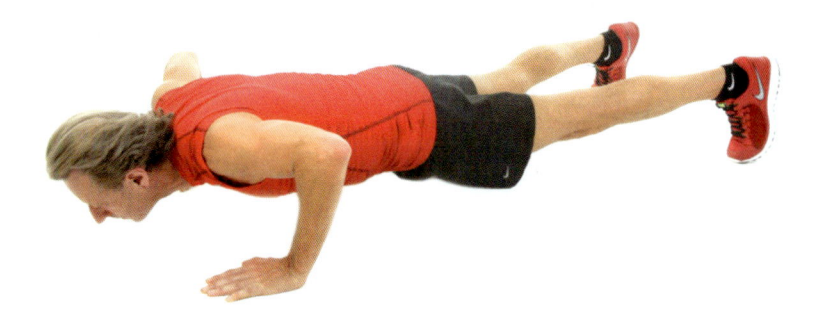

HIIT—HIGH-INTENSITY INTERVAL TRAINING

EXERCISE 3: KNEE TUCK JUMP

Stand with good posture and your knees slightly bent. Jump up high and try to bring your knees into your stomach and place hands on the knees. Land softly and try to repeat this for 40 seconds and then rest for 10 seconds.

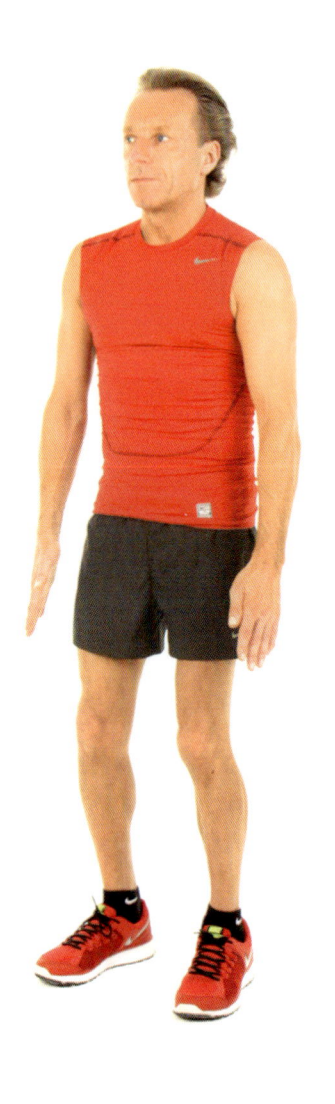

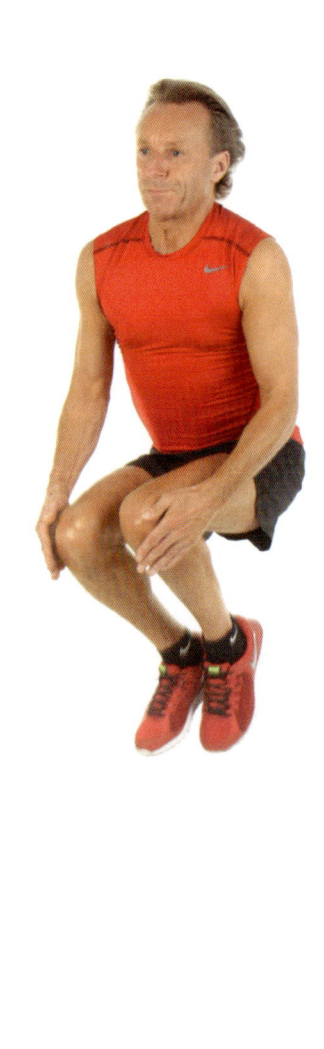

EXERCISE 4: PUSH-UPS

Starting in a full push-up position, slowly lower your chest to the ground, keeping tummy muscles pulled in. Aim for 40 repetitions. If you need to rest, that's fine. Rest for 10 seconds. Come into a kneeling position to give the upper body a little rest. Then finish the remaining repetitions.

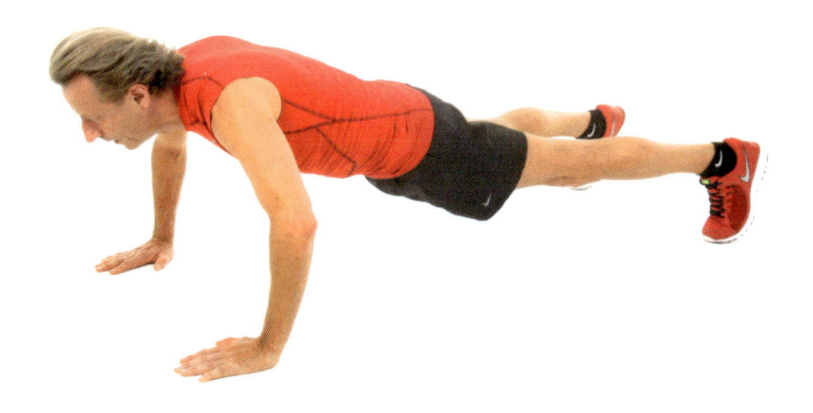

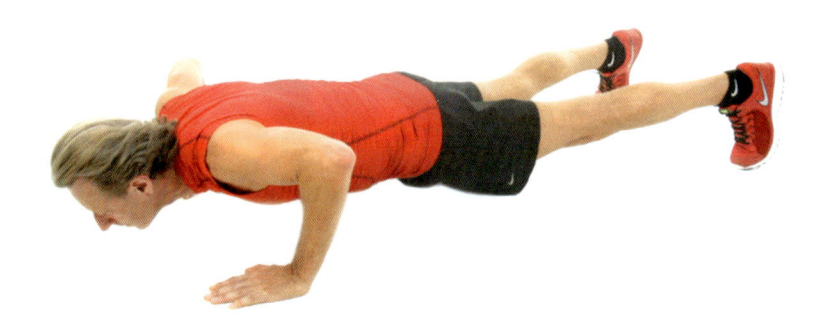

HIIT—HIGH-INTENSITY INTERVAL TRAINING

EXERCISE 7: RIGHT LEG HOP

Hop on your right leg, keeping your upper body straight and landing softly. Do this for 40 seconds and then rest for 10 seconds..

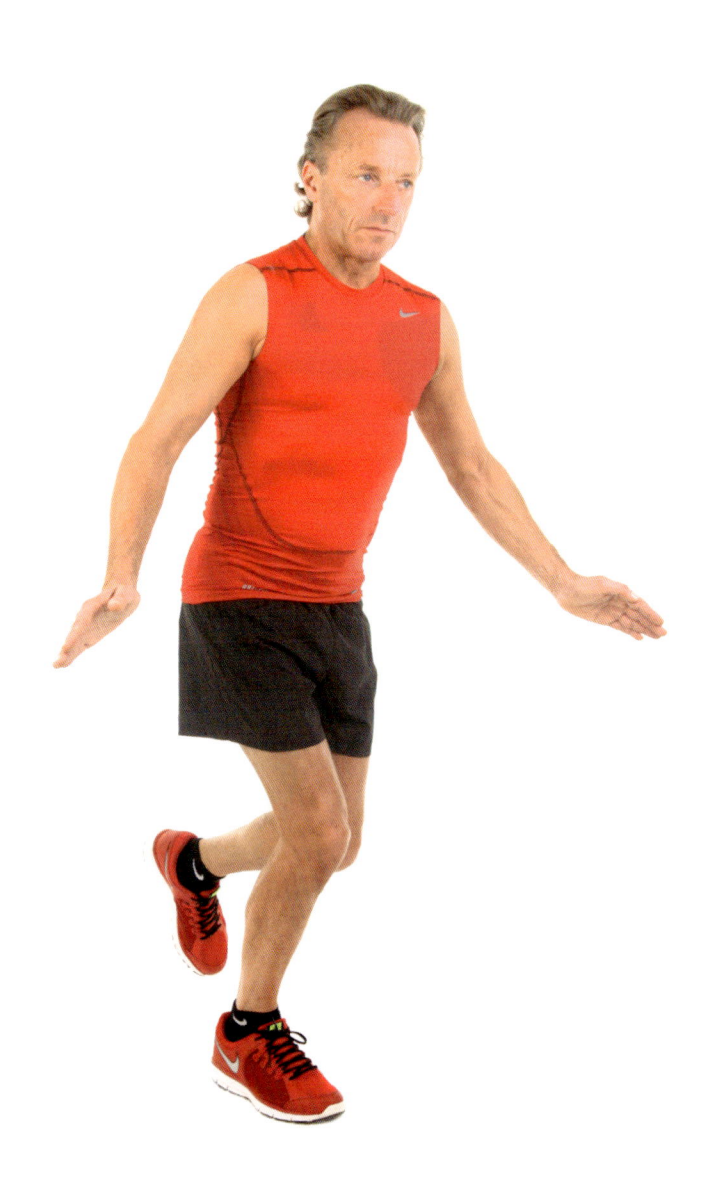

PART II | THE WORKOUTS

EXERCISE 8: PUSH-UPS

Starting in a full push-up position, slowly lower your chest to the ground, keeping tummy muscles pulled in. Aim for 30 repetitions. If you need to rest, that's fine. Rest for 10 seconds. Come into a kneeling position to give the upper body a little rest. Then finish the remaining repetitions.

Complete your cool-down on pages 35-41, and drink a glass of water.

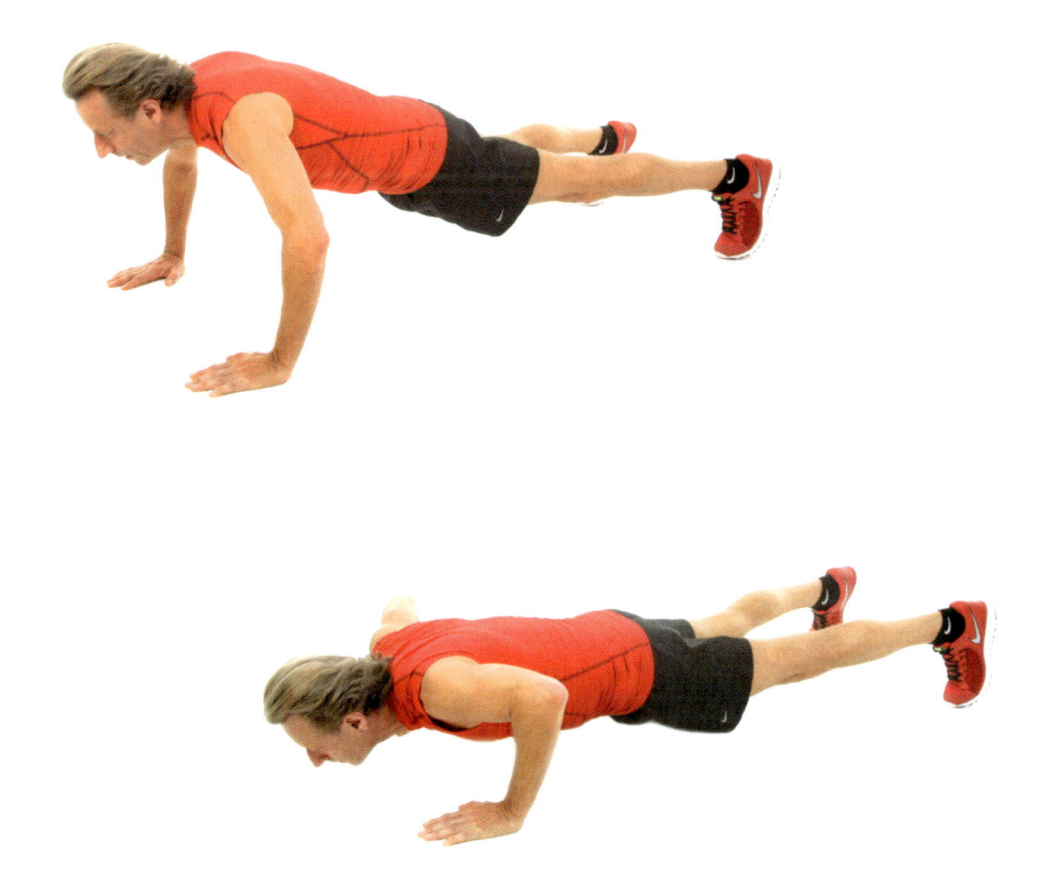

EXERCISE 2: V-KICK ABS

Start in a seated position with your knees bent, both feet off the floor, your arms behind you, and your fingers pointing forward. Keep tummy muscles pulled in and slowly bend your elbows, lowering yourself several inches closer to the ground. At the same time extend legs away from you, hold the position, and then draw the legs back in. Perform 20 repetitions slowly. It is very important throughout the exercise that you constantly engage your abdominal muscles; the lower you go to the ground, the

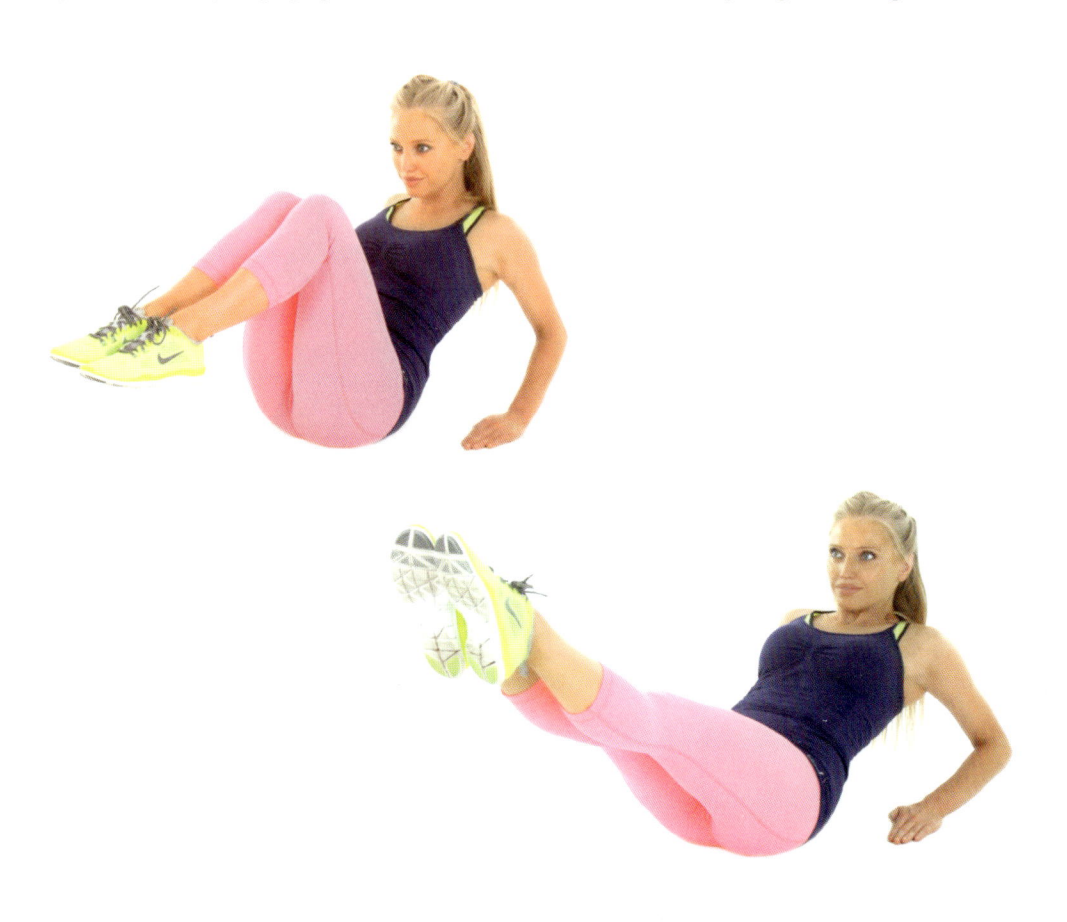

EXERCISE 3: SCISSOR JUMP

Start in an exaggerated march position. Then jump in the air while simultaneously switching the arms and legs. Do this for 50 seconds. Always land softly.

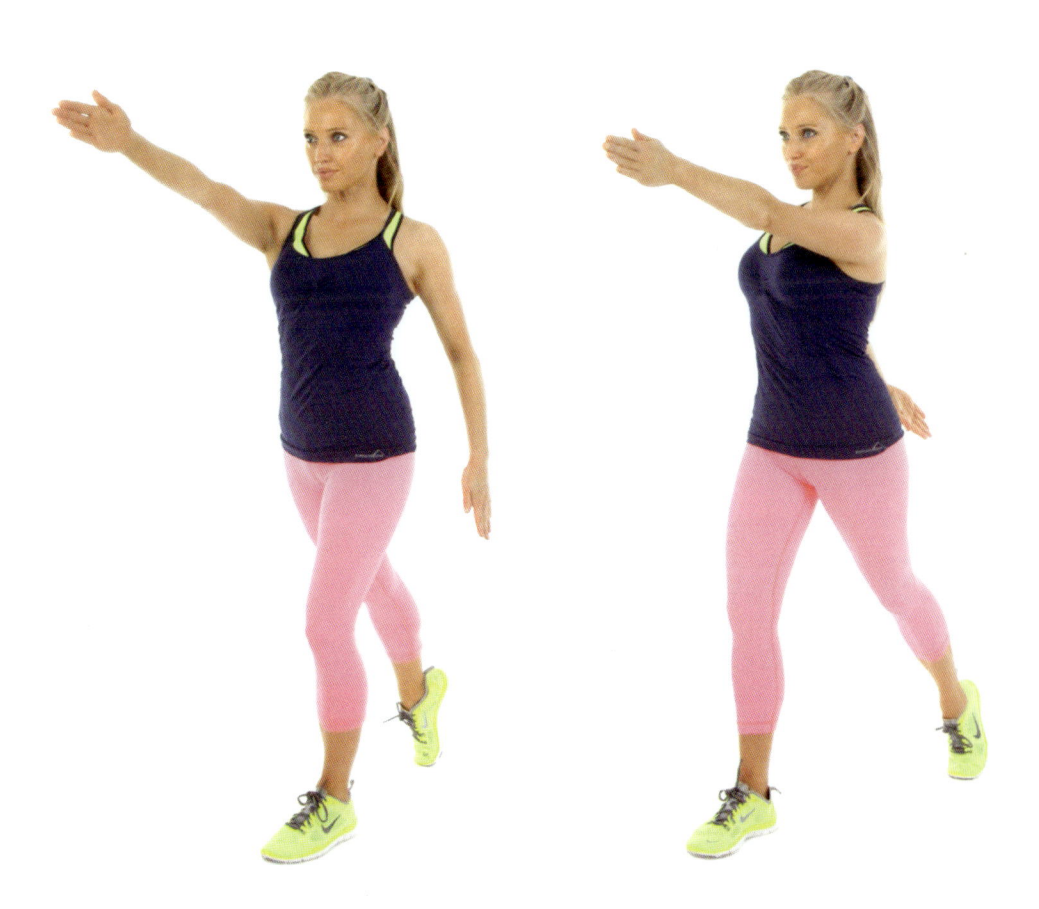

HIIT—HIGH-INTENSITY INTERVAL TRAINING

EXERCISE 4: REACH IT UP ABS

Lie supine on the floor with both legs fully extended and hip-width apart. Place your fingertips on either side of your head and lift your head, and shoulders off the floor. Hold this position and then extend the left arm straight up, trying to touch the right foot. Hold for a second and then change arms, trying to touch the right hand to the left foot. Do 40 repetitions. Make sure you keep the hips and legs perfectly still.

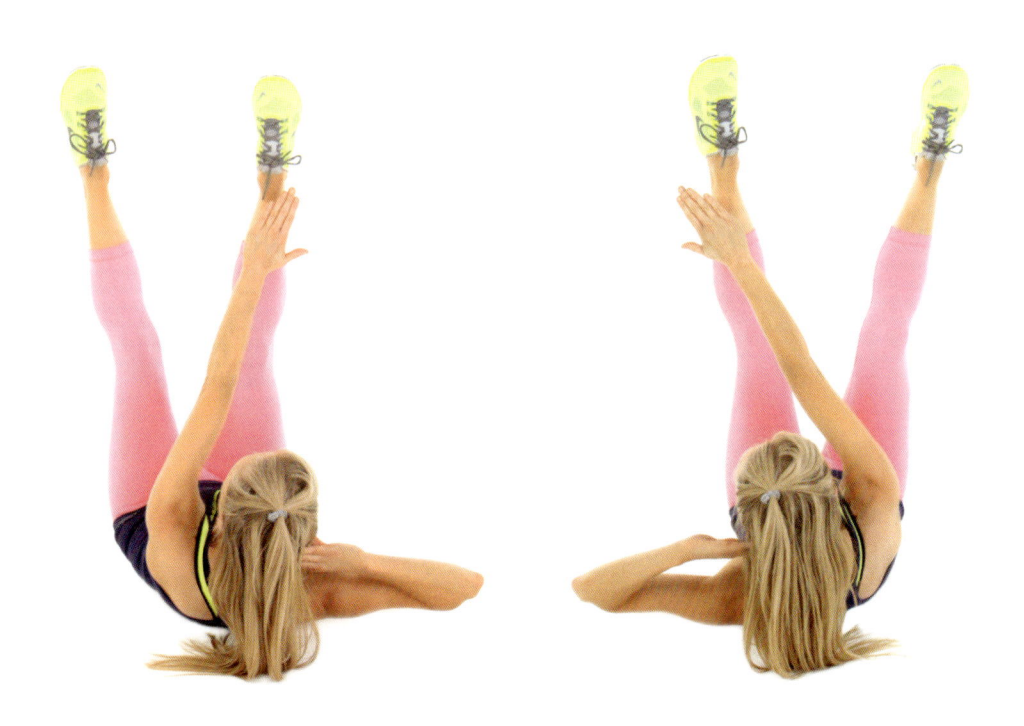

EXERCISE 5: CARDIO PUNCH

Standing in a wide stance with your knees slightly bent and tummy pulled in, punch as hard and as fast as you can from side to side. It is important that you keep the hips still and just focus on the move coming from the upper body. Do this for 50 seconds and then have a 10-second rest period

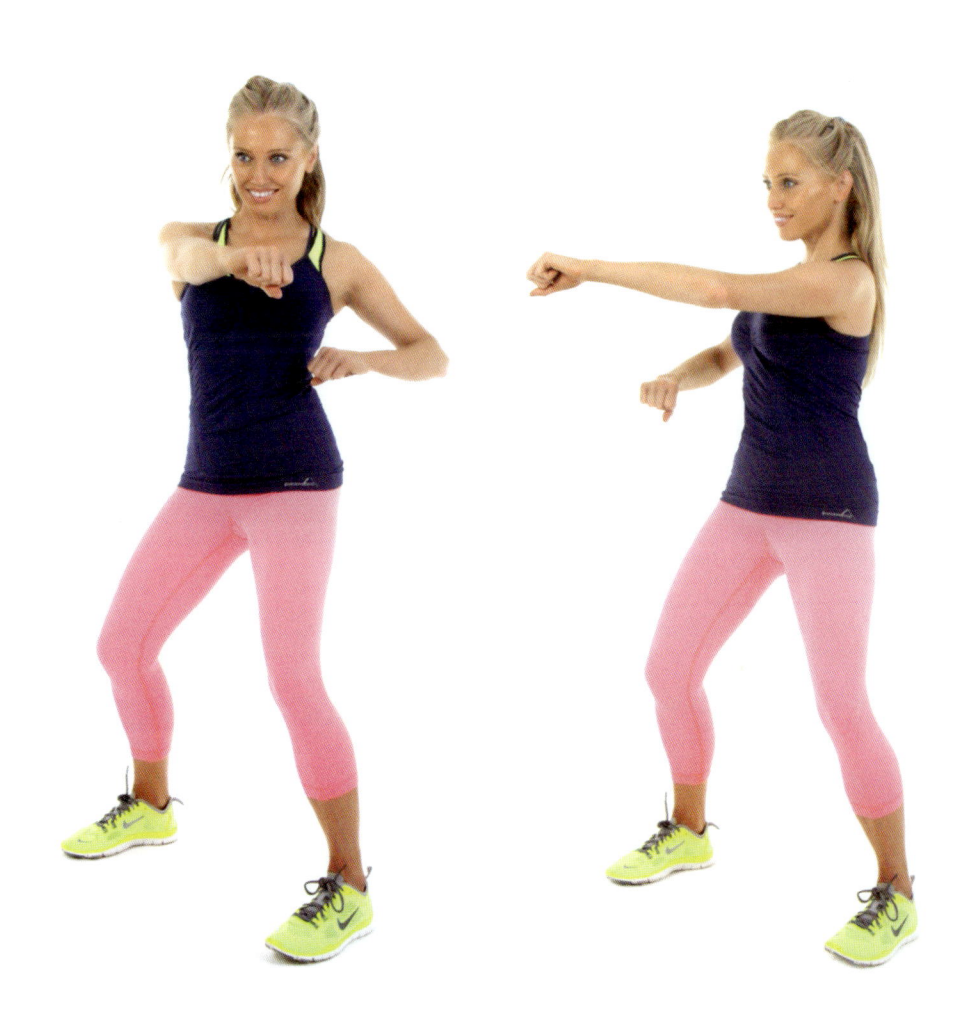

EXERCISE 6: PLANK IT

Get in a plank position with your toes tucked under and elbows directly under your shoulders. Try to keep your body in a straight line, pulling belly button tight toward the spine. Hold this position for 30 seconds.

Repeat the whole routine two times. Then perform all your cool-down stretches on pages 35-41 and drink a glass of water.

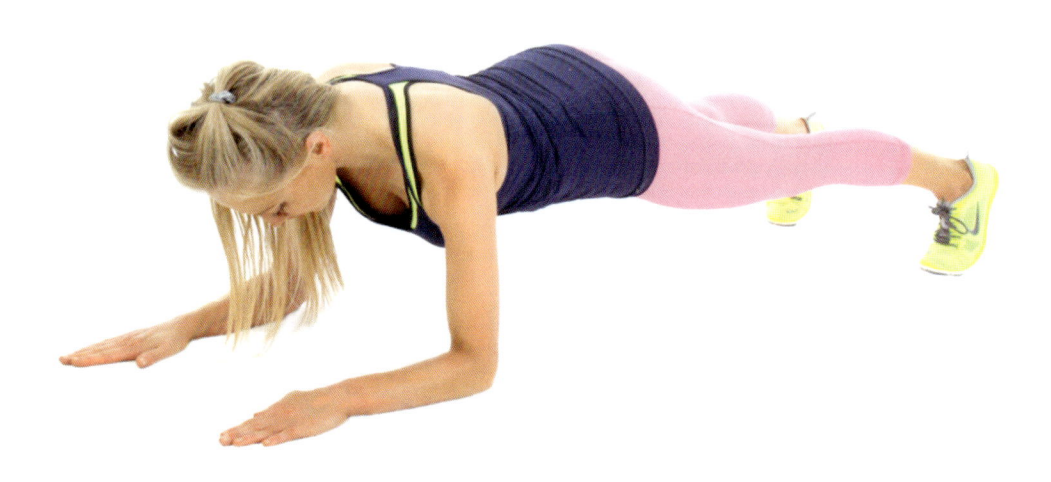

PART II | THE WORKOUTS

18 THE SUPER BODY SCULPTOR HIIT WORKOUT

- Time: Less than 15 MINUTES
- Intensity: HARD
- Timed/Reps: TIMED and REPS
- Planes of Movement: SAGITTAL, FRONTAL, and TRANSVERSE
- Tones: CHEST, BICEPS, TRICEPS, LEGS, BOTTOM, SHOULDERS, OBLIQUES, and ABS
- RPE: 6 to 7

This workout is tough one and works on stripping off excess body fat. The plyometric moves, done for 40-second bursts, will take you to a level 7 (refer to the intensity level chart on page 33). This is the HIIT part of the workout. You then have 10 seconds of recovery before moving straight on to the next move. These exercises work on building power and strength with moves that will sculpt your arms, chest, and abs, giving you that fit, ripped physique.

Always complete the warm-up and cool-down stretches on pages 35-41.

EXERCISE 1: POWER SIDE-TO-SIDE BLAST

Place two dumbbells on the floor several inches apart. Stand by the side of one dumbbell in a deep squat position. Start jumping across them from side to side. Land softly and keep your knees behind the line of your toes. Do this exercise for 40 seconds and then rest for 10 seconds.

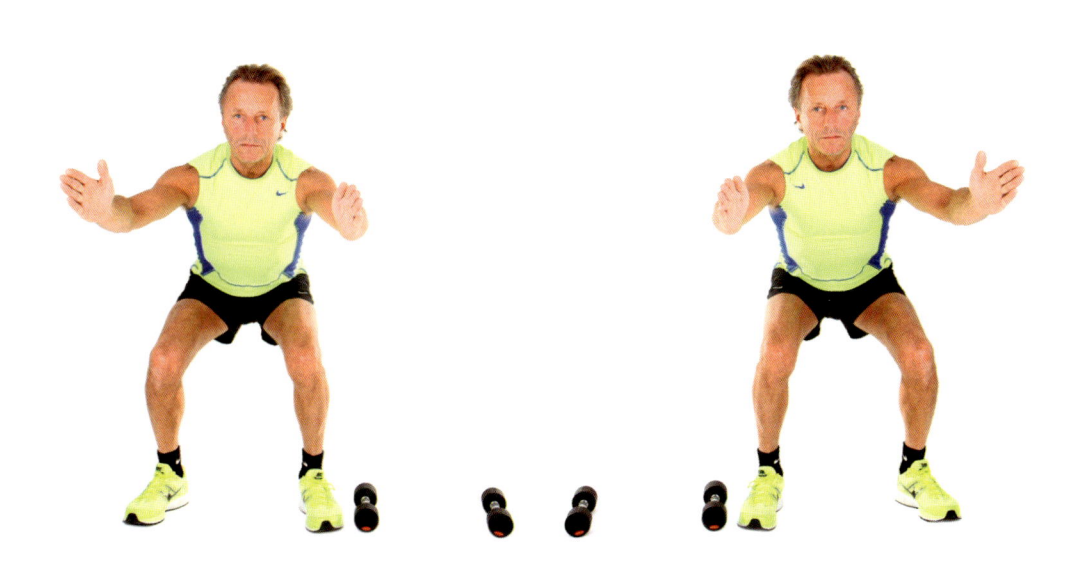

PART II | THE WORKOUTS

EXERCISE 2: IRON MAN PUSH-UP

In a push-up position, place your fingertips together, forming a diamond shape. Slowly lower your chest to the floor, allowing your elbows to point out to the sides. Then slowly push back up. Keep your tummy muscles pulled in tight. Do 20 repetitions slowly.

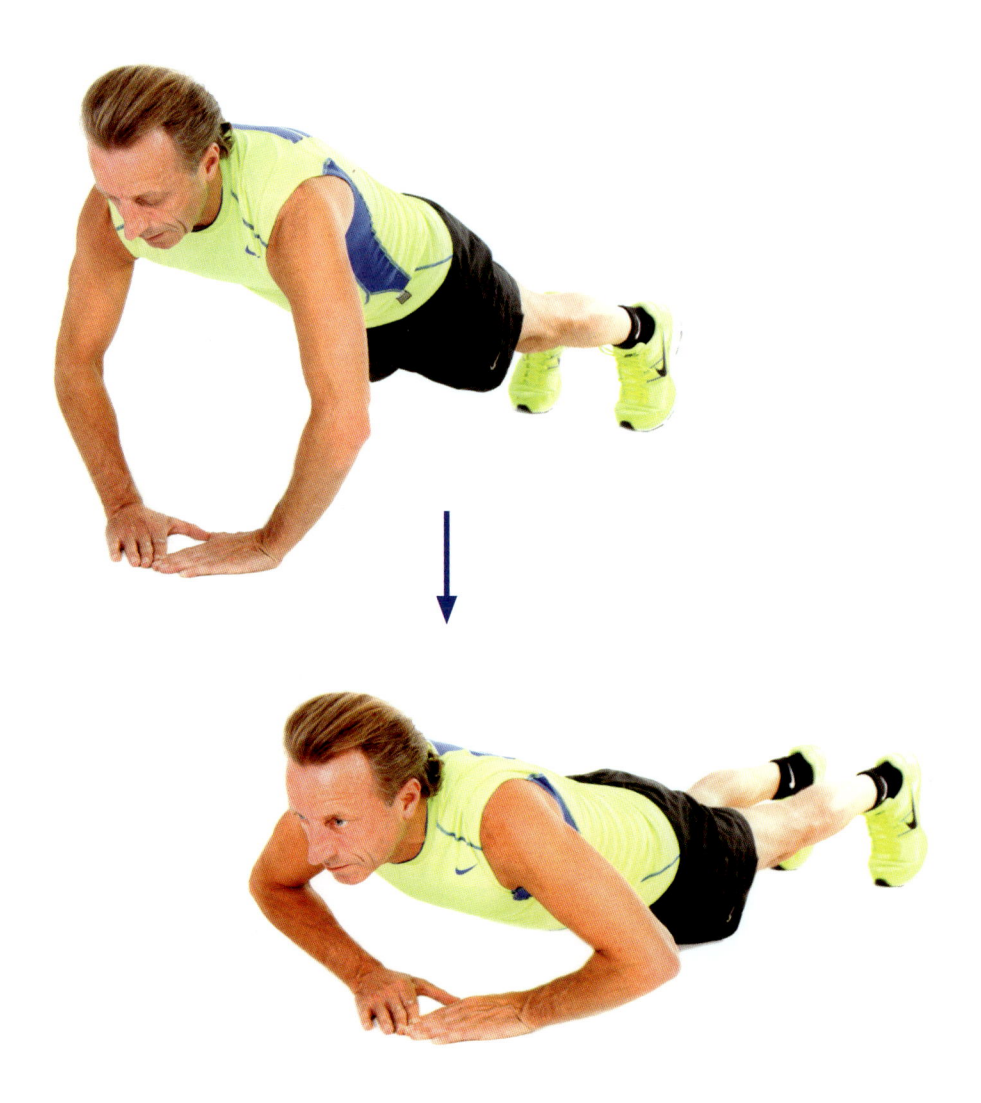

HIIT—HIGH-INTENSITY INTERVAL TRAINING

EXERCISE 3: JUMPING LUNGE

Start in a lunge position with the left leg in front. Jump up, switching legs in the air, and land in a lunge position with the right leg in front. Always keep your upper body straight and land softly. Repeat for 40 seconds and then rest for 10 seconds.

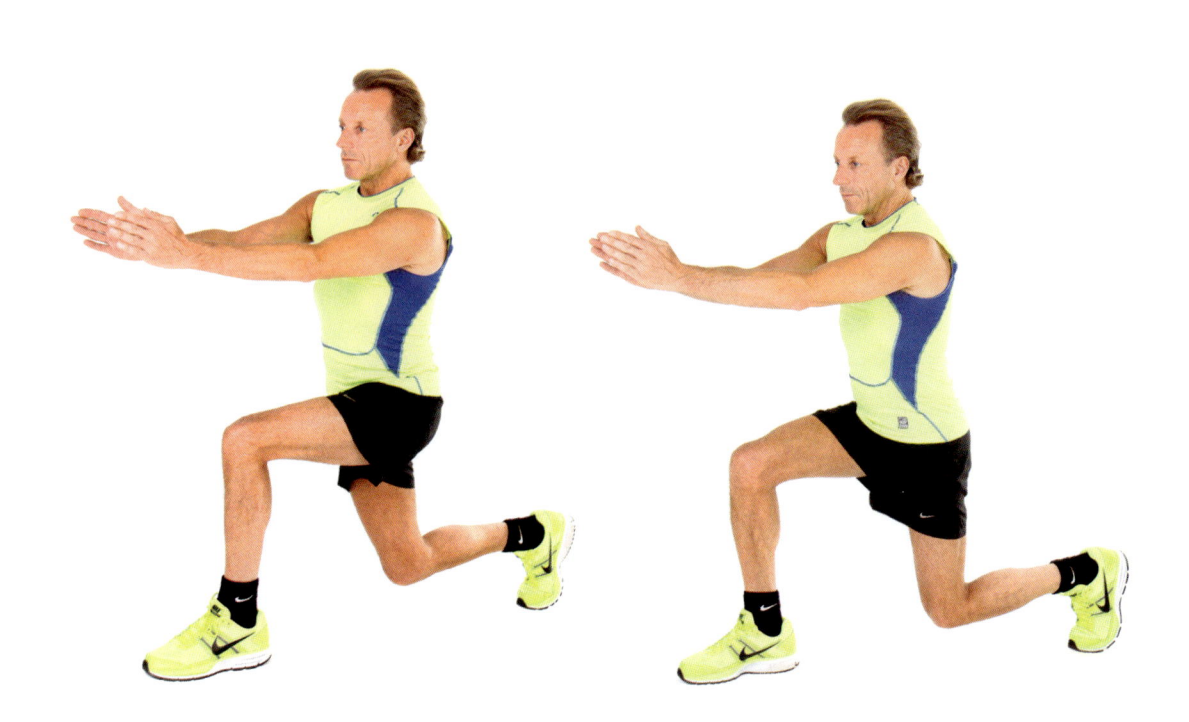

PART II | THE WORKOUTS

EXERCISE 4: ROCK HARD ABS

Lie supine with knees bent and feet flat on the ground, holding your dumbbells (these should not be heavy) on your chest. Pull in your tummy muscles as you sit up and punch your right arm across your body, hold, and then lower back down. Sit back up and punch the left arm across. Keep tummy muscles pulled in tight as you do this. Do 20 repetitions slowly.

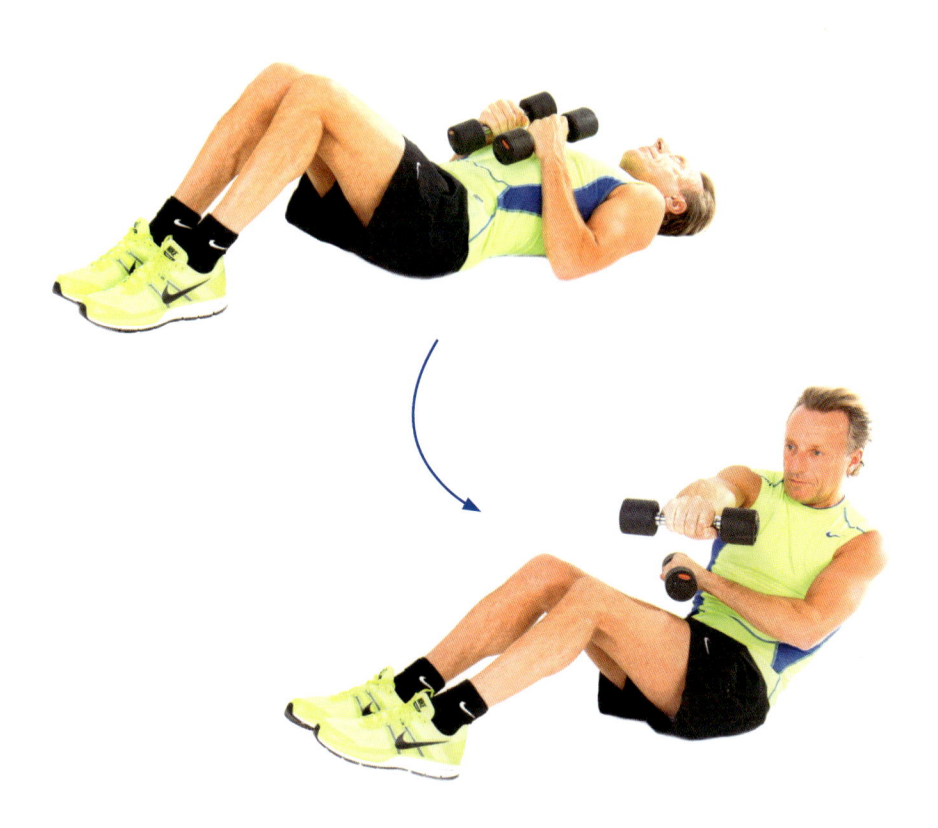

19 THE ULTIMATE HIIT FAT BURNER

- Time: Under 11 MINUTES
- Intensity: MODERATE to HARD
- Timed/Reps: TIMED
- Planes of Movement: SAGITTAL, FRONTAL, and TRANSVERSE
- Tones: BOTTOM, HIPS, THIGHS, CALVES, and ABS
- RPE: 5 to 7

This routine consists of just three moves that work your entire lower body. The benefit of this is that some of the biggest calorie-burning muscles are in the legs and bottom, so the more toned these are, then the more calories you burn. The transitions in each of the exercises also means you get a great cardio workout, so you increase your heart rate. This is what makes it the ultimate fat burner. Before you start, make sure you have completed your warm-up and stretches on pages 35-41.

PART II | THE WORKOUTS

EXERCISE 1: BASKETBALL SIDE STEP

Start in a squat position with your arms bent in front. Staying low, take a big, wide step out to your right. Stay in the low squat, and then jump up high as if you are trying to shoot a basketball. Lift the arms at the same time, and then land back into your squat. Step out to the left and repeat.

Repeat for a total of 50 seconds and then take a 10-second rest period.

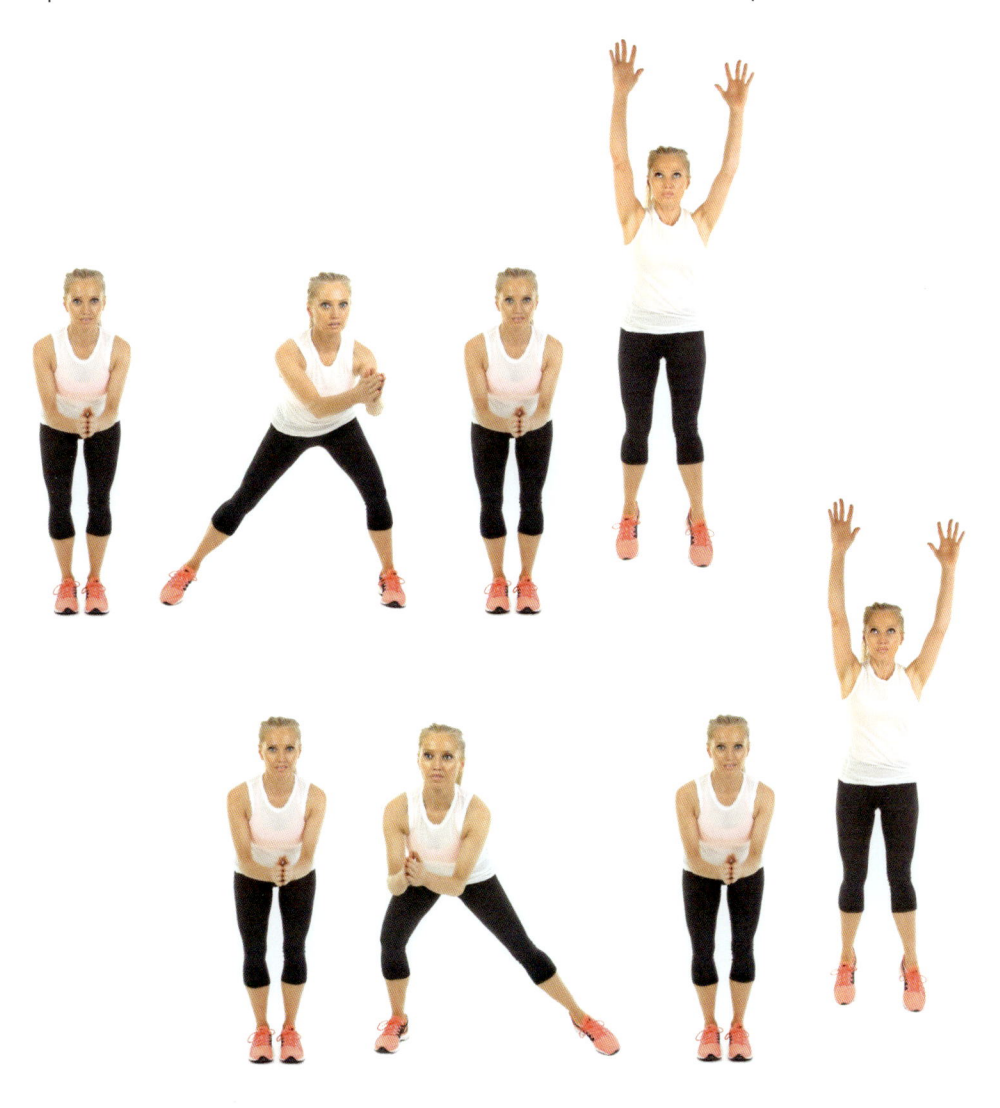

HIIT—HIGH-INTENSITY INTERVAL TRAINING

EXERCISE 2: JUMP SQUATS

Again start in a low squat; then jump up high. Land back in your low squat, and hold the squat position for 10 seconds. Then jump high again. Keep doing this for a total of 50 seconds and take a 10-second rest period.

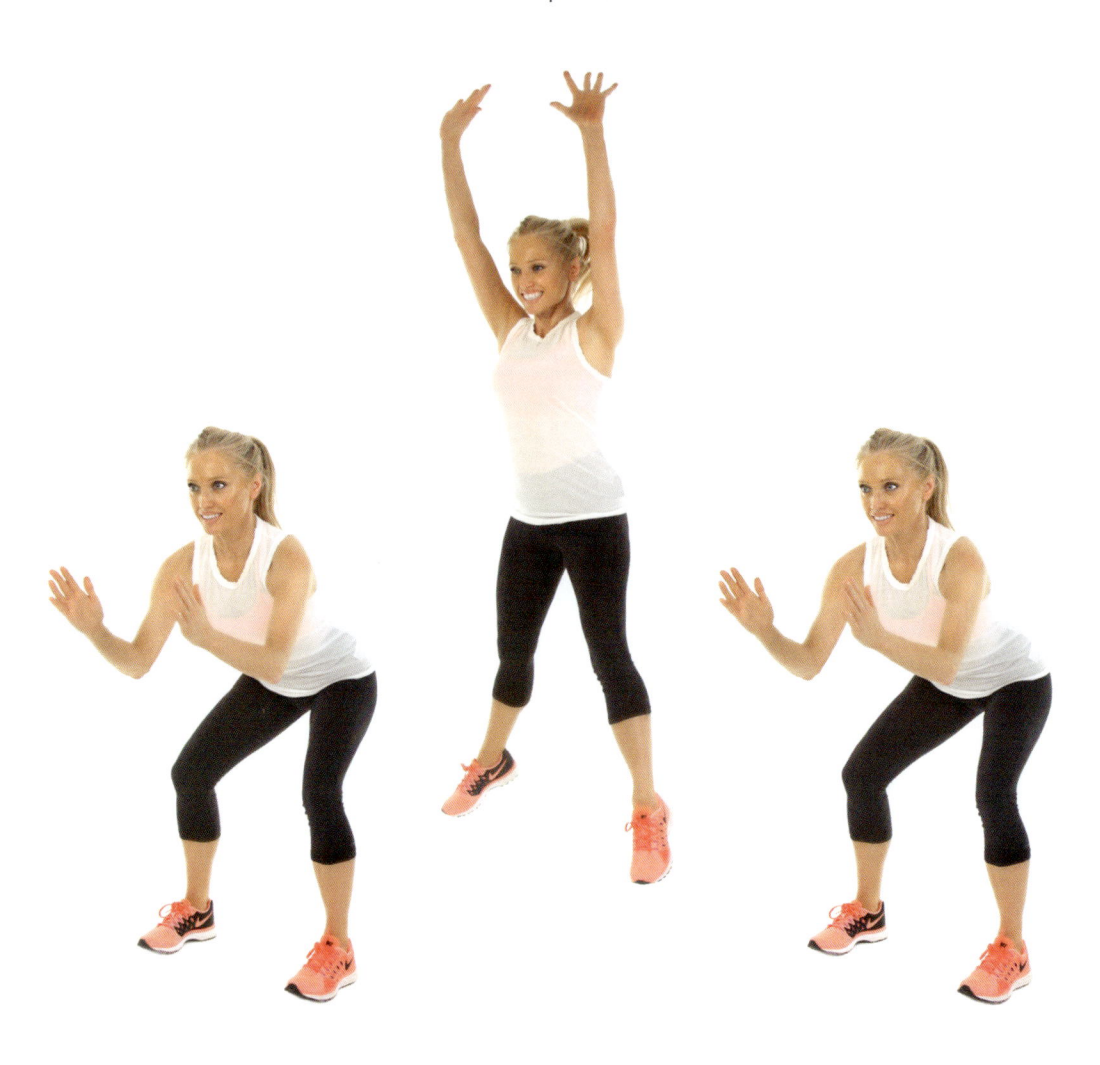

EXERCISE 3: ULTIMATE LEG TONER

Stand with the feet close together and palms together in the center. Slowly lift your left leg out to the side with control. Then lower back to the start position. Now lift the right leg out to the side, trying to lift it as high as you can without twisting your body. Make sure the supporting knee is always slightly bent and keep tummy muscles pulled in throughout. Repeat for a total of 50 seconds and then take a 10-second rest period.

Have a 20-second rest period and then repeat the routine another two times. At the end finish off with a glass of water and do your cool-down stretches on pages 35-41.

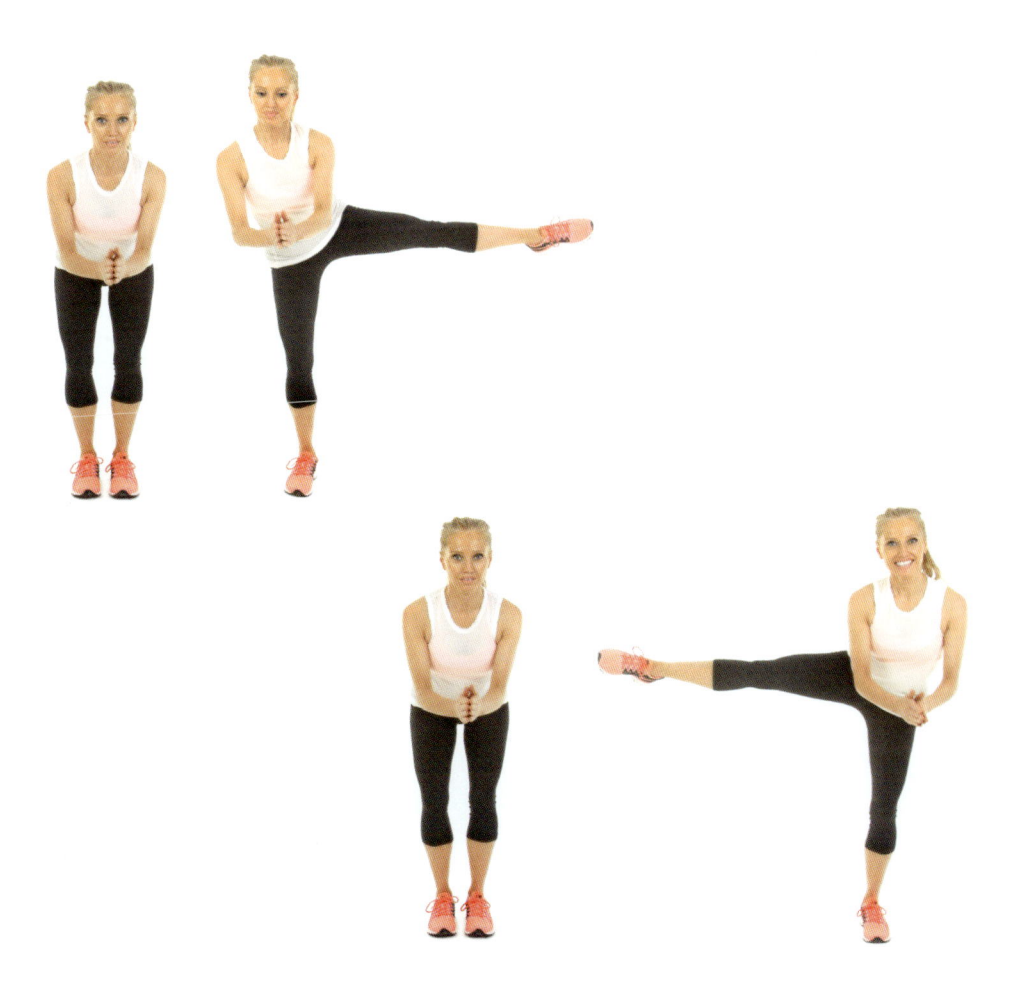

20 THE WALKING HIIT WORKOUT

- Time: 14 MINUTES
- Intensity: MODERATE to HARD
- Timed/Reps: TIMED
- Planes of Movement: SAGITTAL and FRONTAL
- Tones: ABS, WAIST, LEGS, BOTTOM, HIPS, ARMS, and CALVES
- RPE: 5 to 7

Walking is one of the most natural exercises we can do, and this low-impact move helps to tone and sculpt you all over. By adding this HIIT workout, you can burn off excess calories and increase your general fitness. Walking is a great way to tone your legs, bottom, abs, and arms; plus if you add any hills to your workout, you will then work those legs and bottom muscles even harder, which is great for seeing results quickly.

PART II | THE WORKOUTS

15-MINUTE WALKING HIIT WORKOUT

- 1 minute brisk pace: Level 5
- 30 seconds shorter stride but faster pace: Level 6
- 20 seconds normal stride but fastest pace: Level 7
- 10 seconds gentle walk: Level 4
- REPEAT 7 TIMES
- Then finish with 40 star jumps (page 95).

TIP:
Always walk with good posture and imagine you are walking along a tightrope. This ensures you walk with good posture and in good alignment.

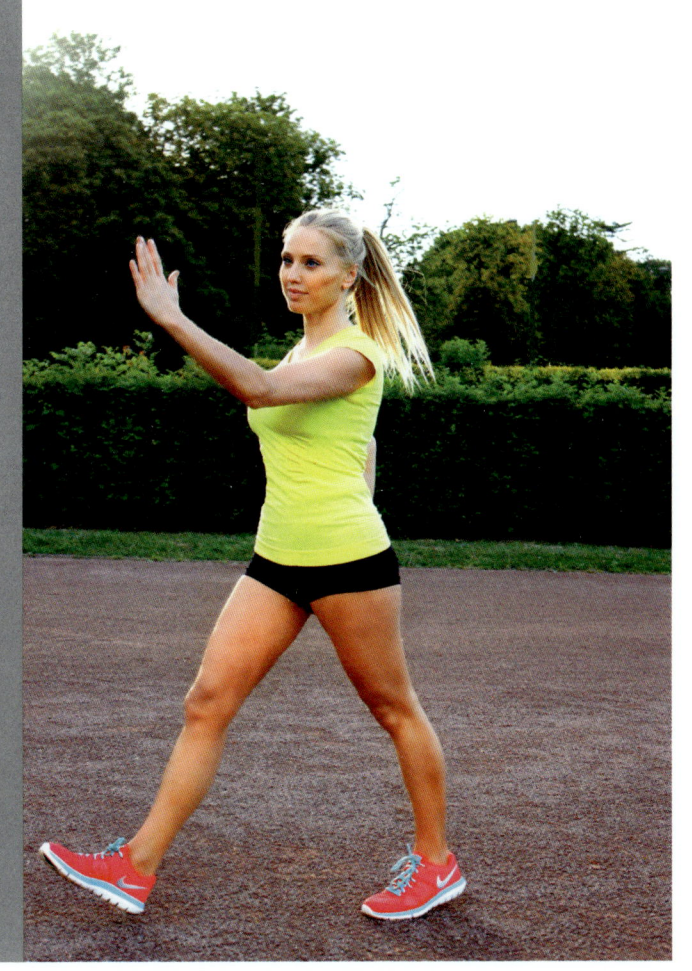

21 RUNNING HIIT WORKOUT

- Time: 15 MINUTES
- Intensity: MODERATE to HARD
- Timed/Reps: TIMED
- Planes of Movement: SAGITTAL, FRONTAL, and TRANSVERSE
- Tones: ABS, WAIST, CORE, LEGS, and BOTTOM
- RPE: 5 to 7

Improve your running endurance and speed with this HIIT workout. The shorter bursts of higher intensity will help to increase your pace and improve your running stamina. At the end of the workout, I recommend you to do 20 power side-to-side blasts (page 102) because this provides you with a powerful plyometric move that will help build power in your legs and also engage the extra plane of movement. When you get fitter, you can add the 15-minute routine provided next to your running. Using slight inclines as the hills are a great way to build power in the lower body, which ultimately helps with your speed.

PART II | THE WORKOUTS

THE 15-MINUTE ROUTINE

- 2 minutes and 30 seconds running at a normal pace: Level 5
- 20 seconds sprinting as fast as you can: Level 7
- 10 seconds gentle jogging: Level 5
- REPEAT 5 TIMES
- Finish with 40 POWER SIDE-TO-SIDE BLASTS (page 102).

> **RUNNING TIP**
> Breathe through your nose and mouth to make sure you get plenty of oxygen to your muscles while running. When running at a slower pace, focus on taking deep belly breaths as this will help prevent any side stitches.

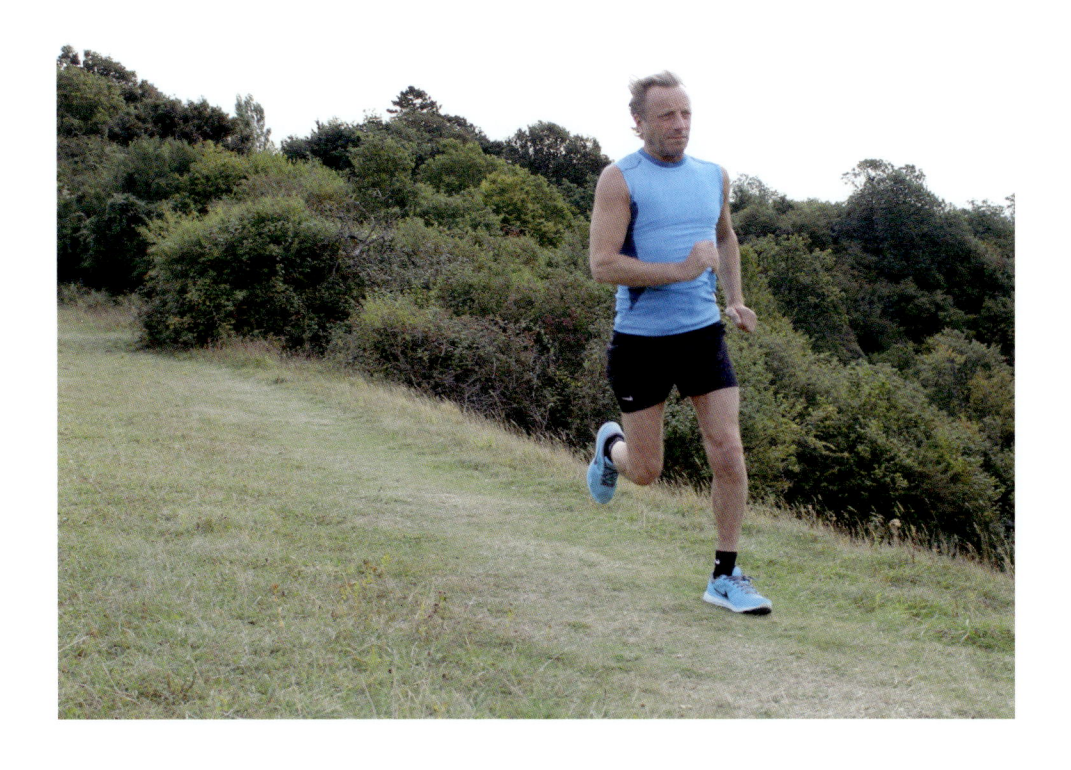

HIIT—HIGH-INTENSITY INTERVAL TRAINING

22 THE FREE WEIGHTS HIIT WORKOUT

- Time: 15 MINUTES
- Intensity: MODERATE to HARD
- Timed/Reps: TIMED and REPS
- Planes of Movement: SAGITTAL and TRANSVERSE
- Tones: BICEPS, SHOULDERS, OBLIQUES, CHEST, TRICEPS, LEGS, BOTTOM, and ABS
- RPE: 5 to 7.5

This workout proves that HIIT is not all about cardio! You can get amazing results by doing a mix of cardio and free weights, and the benefit of both these styles of training is that they are both high fat burners. Mixing them together not only helps build a stronger muscular body but also helps strip off excess body fat by elevating your resting metabolic rate (the amount of calories your body burns). It stays elevated for hours after your workout. Before you perform your workout, make sure you complete your warm-up on pages 35-41. For the free weights, I recommend you use a weight that you can lift for at least 8 to 12 repetitions before it feels challenging, so a good guide is to find the weight that hits that challenge point. If you feel challenged after a few repetitions, the weight is too heavy, and if you feel you could keep going after 25 repetitions, the weight is too light.

PART II | THE WORKOUTS

EXERCISE 1: HIGH KNEES IN PLACE

Running in place, try to get your knees high, pumping through with your arms. Keep your back straight and land softly. Do this for 60 seconds and then gently march in place for 10 seconds.

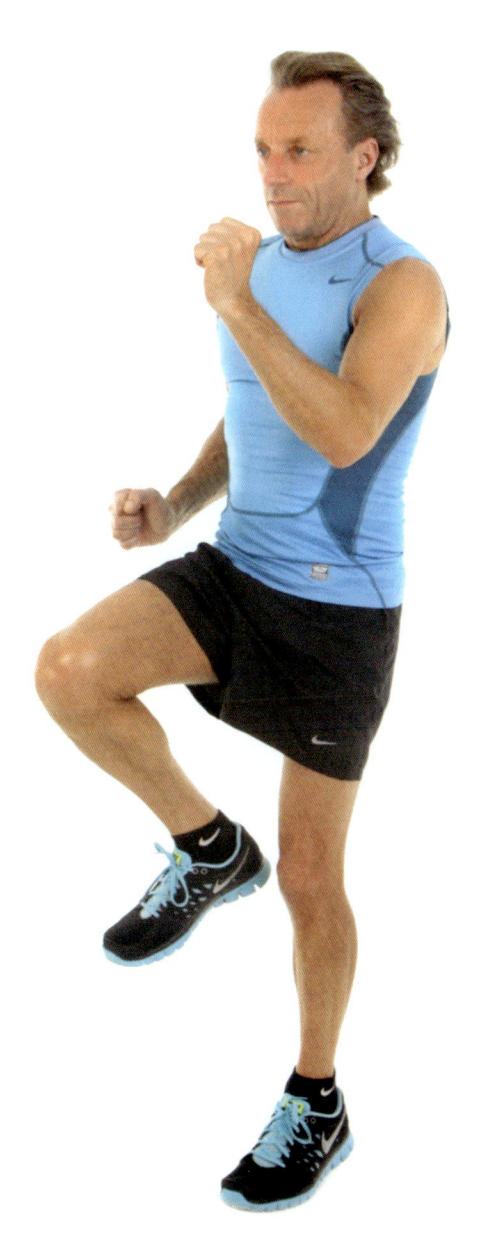

EXERCISE 4: WEIGHTED SIDE BENDS

Hold your free weights on either side of your body. Slowly bend to one side, lowering the weight toward your knee while bringing the other weight up close to your chest. Hold for a second and then slowly lower back down, alternating from side to side. It is important that you keep your knees soft and your tummy muscles pulled in. Don't lean forward or backward. Aim to do 22 repetitions.

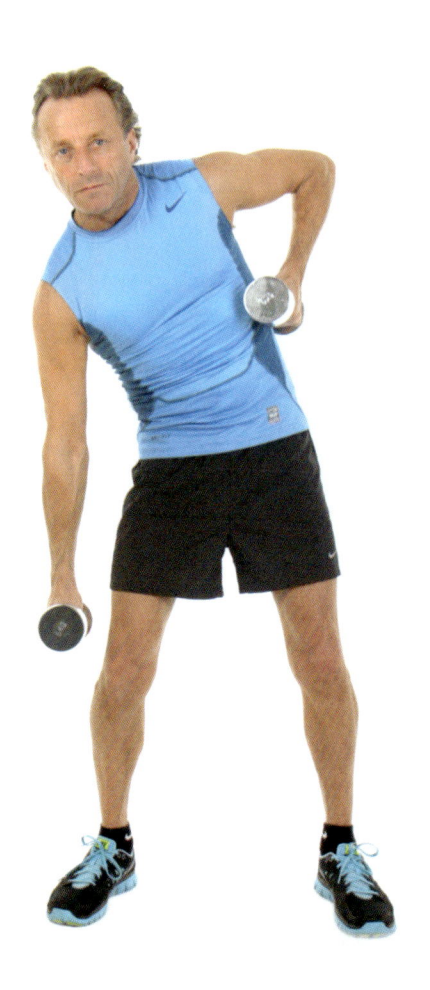

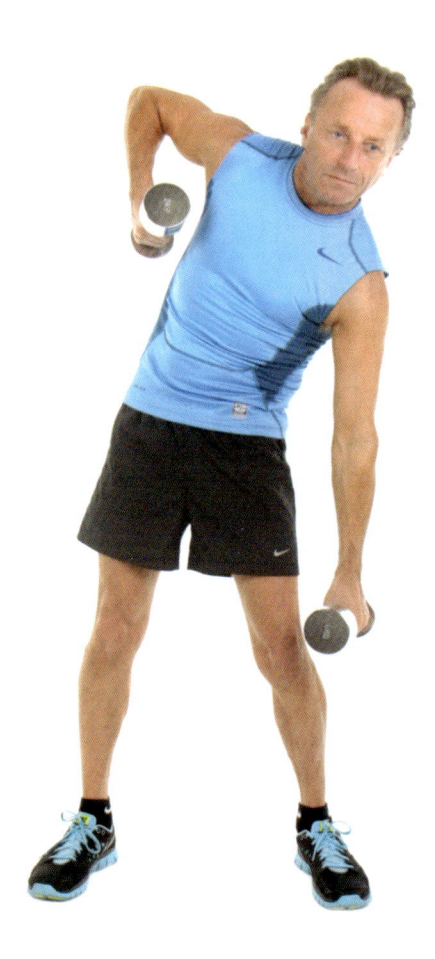

EXERCISE 5: HIGH KNEES IN PLACE

Running in place, try to get your knees high, pumping through with your arms. Keep your back straight and land softly. Do this for 40 seconds and then gently march in place for 10 seconds.

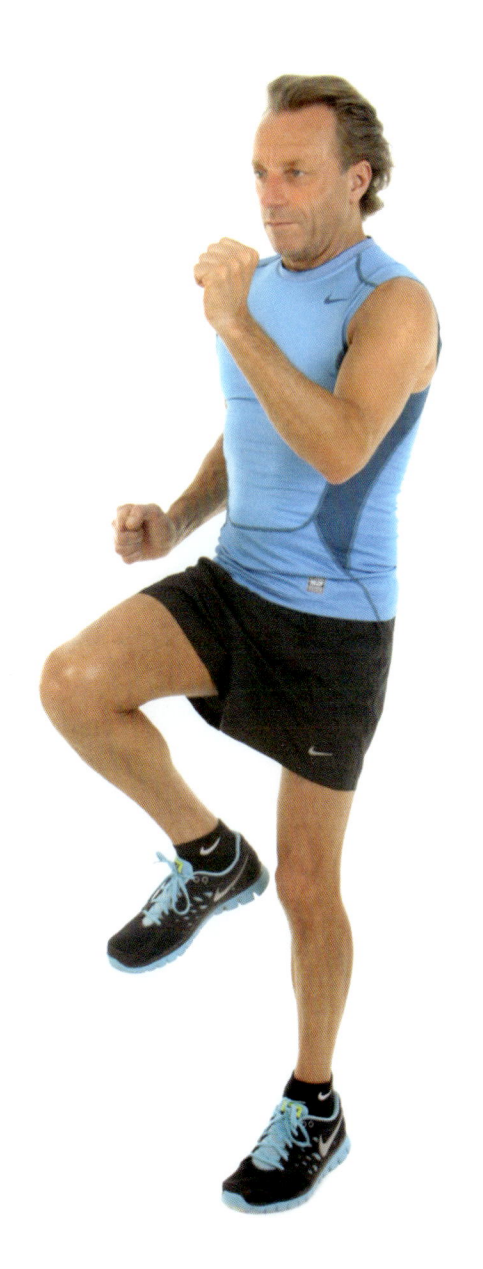

EXERCISE 8: FREE WEIGHT LUNGE

Stand with good posture and your arms down by your sides. Now lunge forward on your left leg while at the same time bringing both your arms up to you toward your chest. Hold and then push back off the left foot and come up to standing and straighten the arms. Then lunge with right foot, again performing a biceps curl with the weights. Aim to do 20 alternating repetitions.

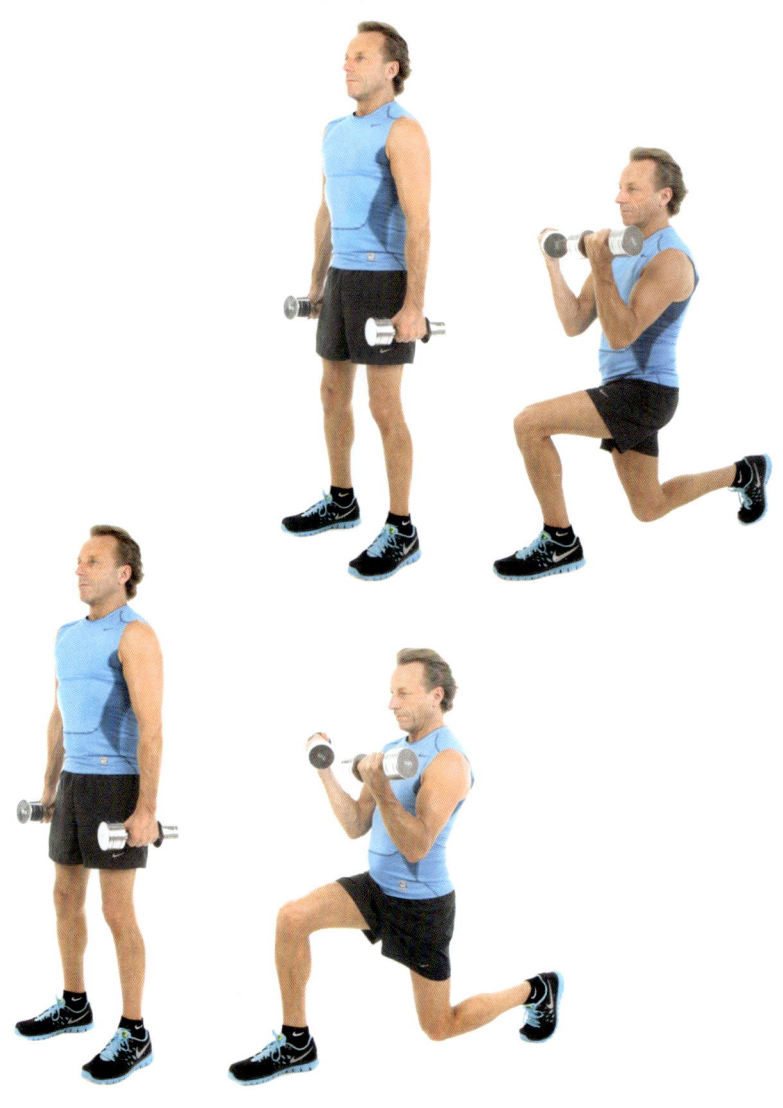

EXERCISE 9: HIGH KNEES IN PLACE

Running in place, try to get your knees high, pumping through with your arms. Keep your back straight and land softly. Do this for 20 seconds and then gently march in place for 10 seconds.

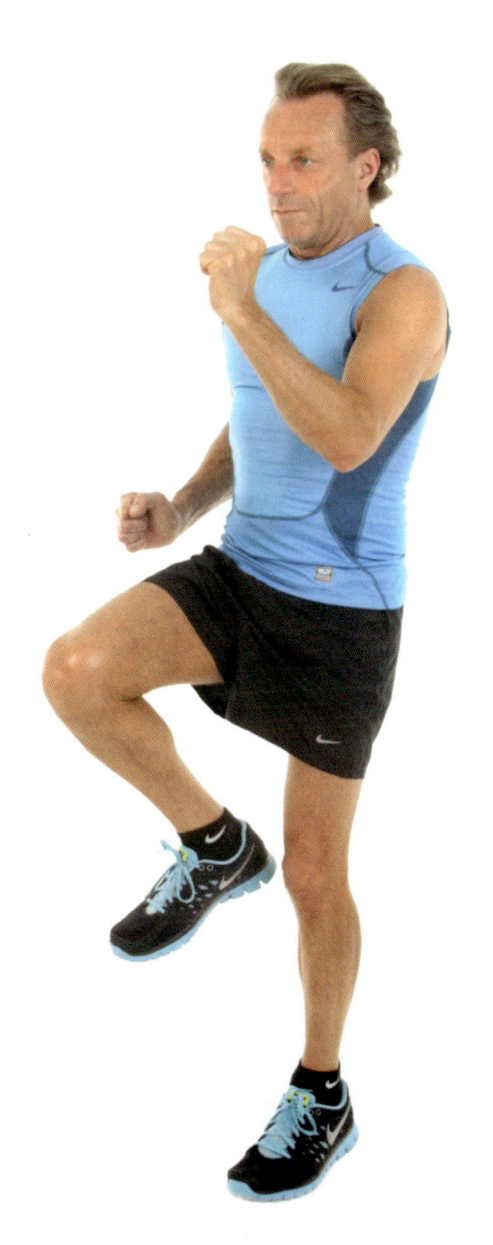

HIIT—HIGH-INTENSITY INTERVAL TRAINING

EXERCISE 1: LEFT LEG HOP SKIP

Skip by doing a hopping skip on your left leg for 30 seconds. If you are new to skipping, then stick with a basic skip.

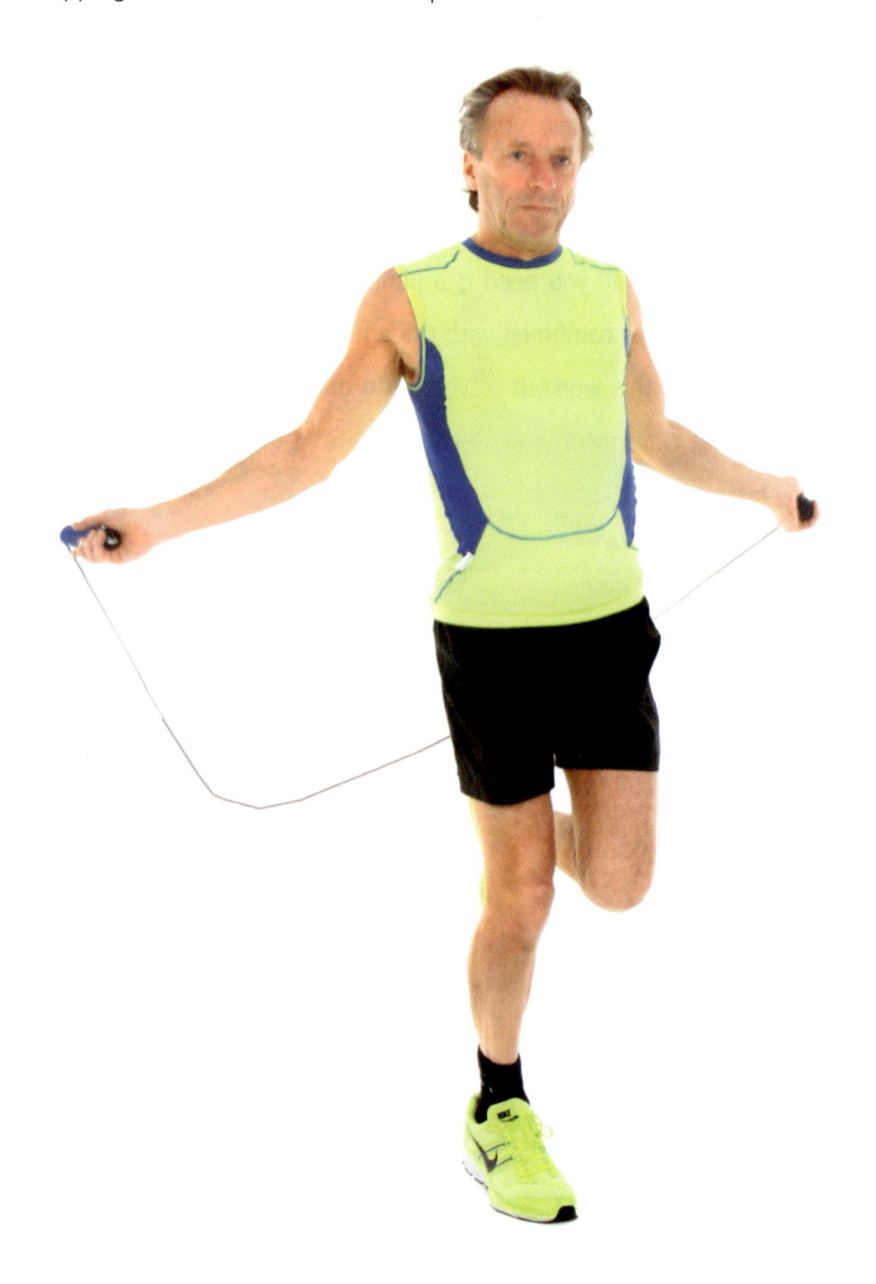

PART II | THE WORKOUTS

EXERCISE 2: SQUAT JUMP ROPE

Lay the skipping rope on the floor and stand behind it. Come into a squat position and then jump over the rope, landing in a deep squat. Then jump back over the rope. Do 30 repetitions.

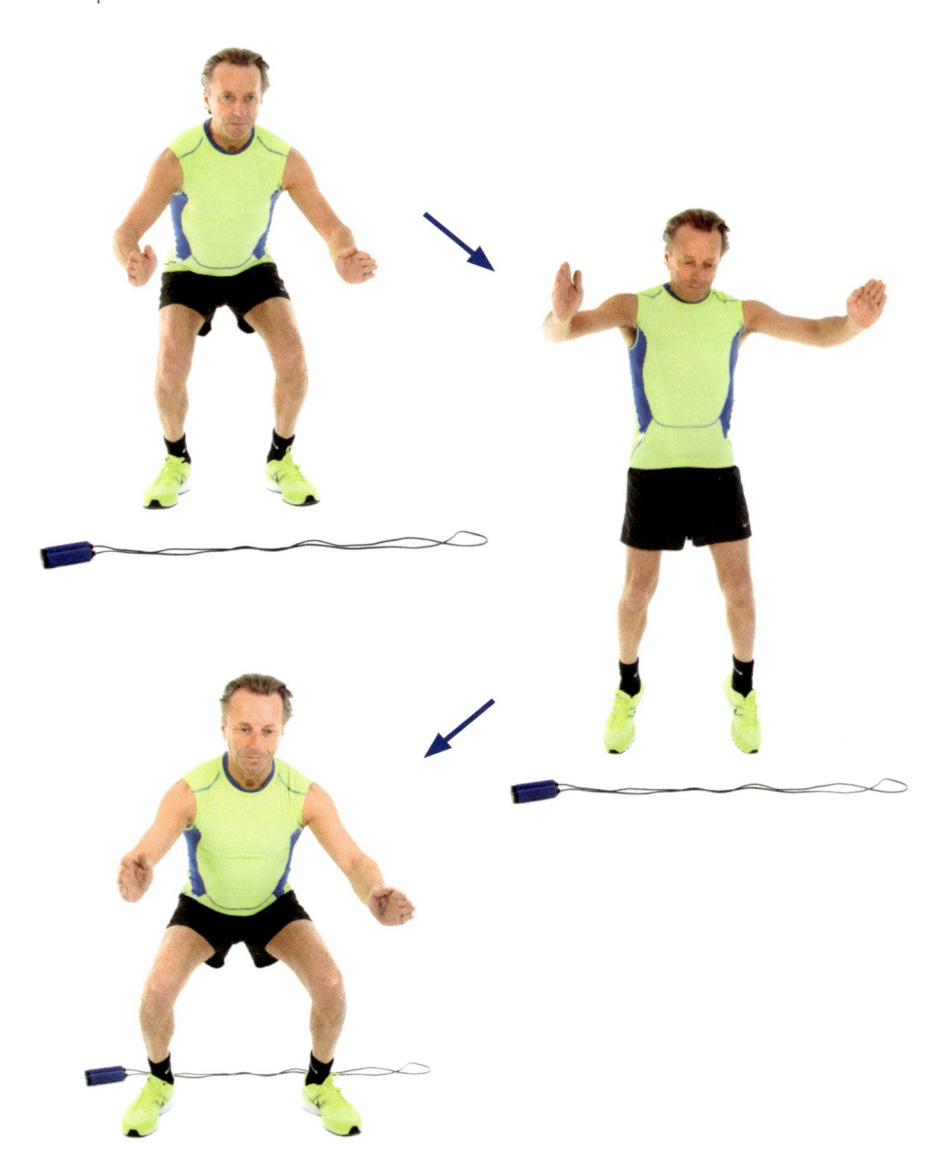

EXERCISE 5: RIGHT LEG HOP SKIP

Do skipping hops on the right foot. Aim to do this for 30 seconds. If you are new to skipping, then stick with a basic skip.

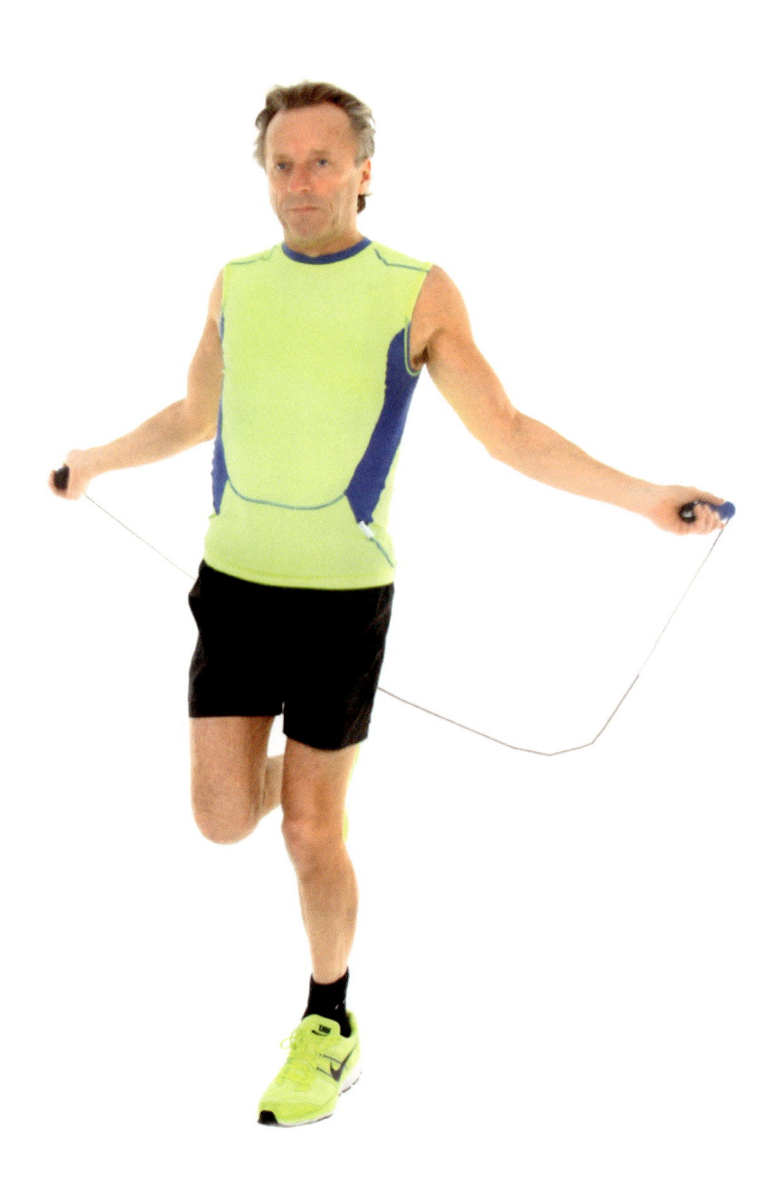

PART II | THE WORKOUTS

EXERCISE 6: ULTIMATE AB MOVE

Lie supine with legs extended and jump rope wrapped around feet. Hold onto both ends of the rope, wrapping around your hands until the rope has tension. Now lift your head and shoulders off floor and pull the rope from side to side, keeping your head and shoulders off the floor. Do 30 repetitions.

Repeat the routine once more but reduce each exercise by 10, so knock off 10 seconds or 10 repetitions. Then repeat, again knocking off another 10 seconds or 10 repetitions. Then perform your cool-down and stretches; see pages 35-41.

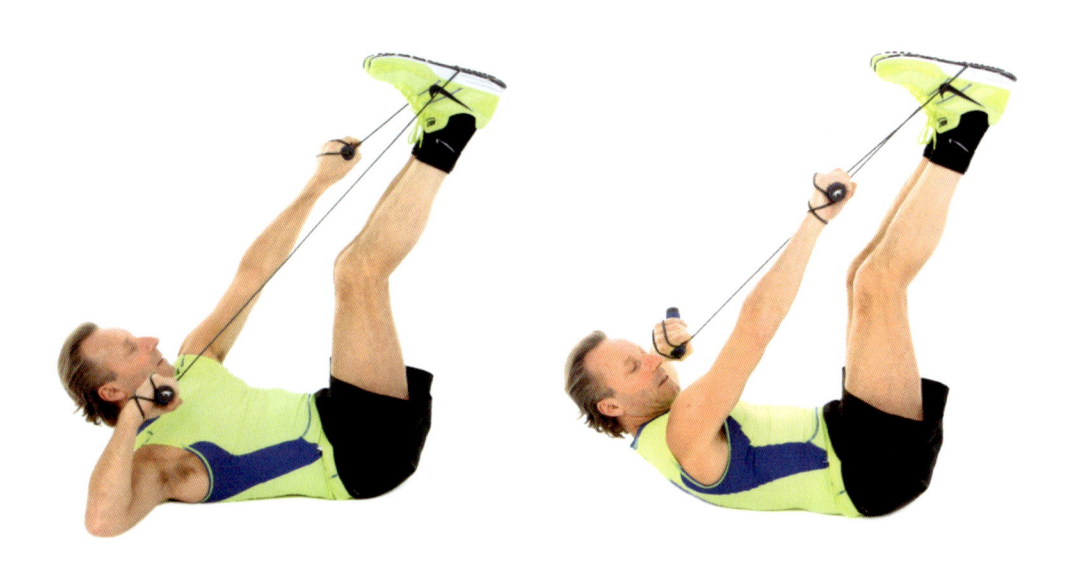

HIIT—HIGH-INTENSITY INTERVAL TRAINING

EXERCISE 2: SHAPE YOUR BOTTOM LIFT

Start in a narrow squat position with your arms bent. Hold this position and then extend up by pushing your arms directly overhead and squeezing one leg out behind you. Hold for a second, really squeezing the bottom of the lifted leg tight. Then come back to the start position and repeat on the opposite leg. Do 40 repetitions of these.

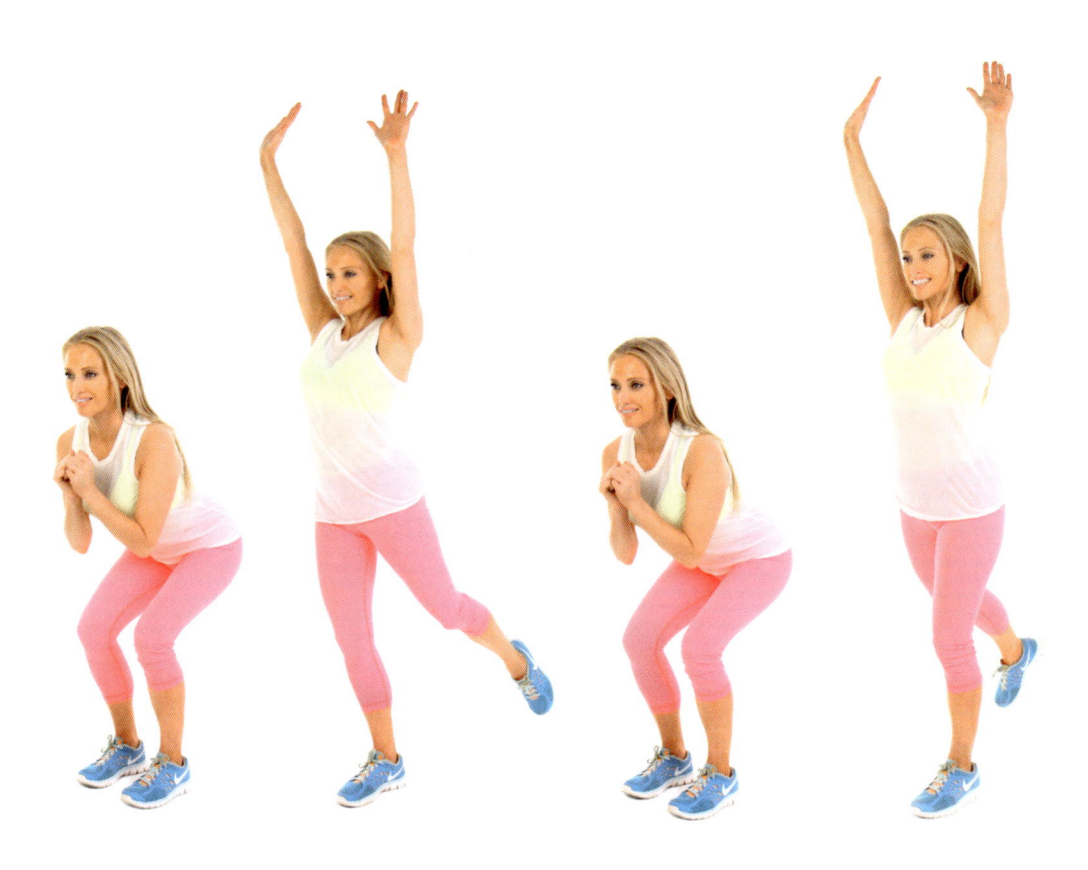

PART II | THE WORKOUTS

EXERCISE 3: JEAN CURTSY

Standing with good posture, feet hip-width apart and arms crossed, slowly curtsy to one side by taking one leg out behind you and then bending through your knees, still keeping the upper body straight. Hold and then return to the start position. Do 20 repetitions on one leg and then do another 20 repetitions on the other leg.

So if you are desperate to feel fab in your skinny jeans, then you could repeat this routine two to three times, and always finish with your cool-down on pages 35-41.

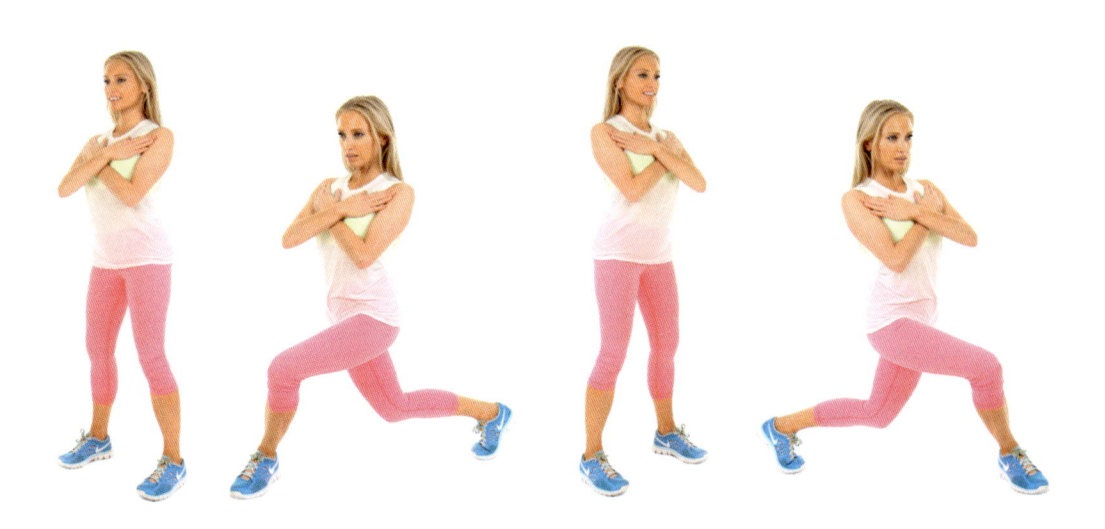

25 THE CALORIE-BURNING CHAIR HIIT WORKOUT

- Time: Under 10 MINUTES
- Intensity: MODERATE to HARD
- Timed/Reps: TIMED and REPS
- Planes of Movement: SAGITTAL, FRONTAL, and TRANSVERSE
- Tones: INNER and OUTER THIGHS, BOTTOM, ABS, ARMS, WAIST, LEGS, and BUST
- RPE: 5 to 7

All you need for this workout is a chair or a sturdy surface; I do recommend that you place the chair against a wall to ensure it stays firmly in place. The seven moves are going to give you a full-body toning workout, and using the chair will help increase your calorie burning. Also always use a great range of movement with each exercise which helps you get amazing results. Before you start, do your warm-up on page 35.

PART II | THE WORKOUTS

EXERCISE 1: STEP IT UP

Stand facing the chair. Step up, ensuring both feet are firmly placed on the chair, hold for a second, and then step back down. Lead with the left leg for 30 seconds, and then lead with the right leg for the another 30 seconds. Constantly maintain good posture and keep your tummy pulled in.

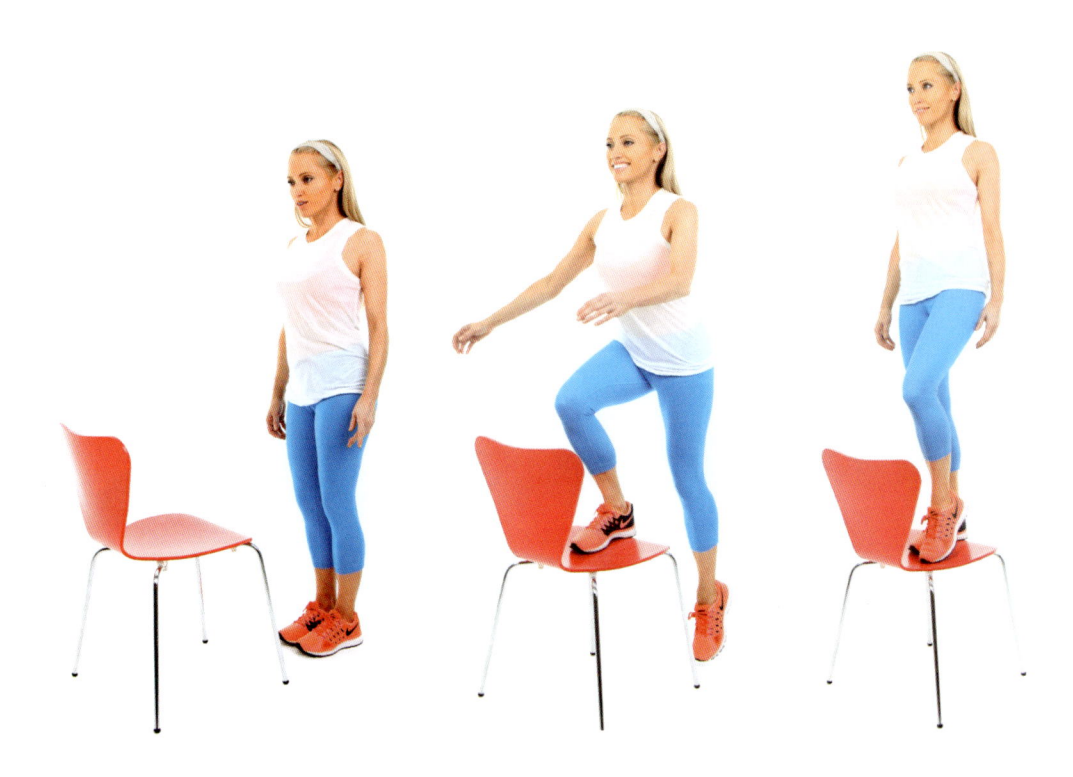

139

HIIT—HIGH-INTENSITY INTERVAL TRAINING

EXERCISE 2: CALORIE RUN

Lean into your chair so your hips are dropped and hands firmly placed on the chair. Place the chair against a wall to ensure it cannot slip. Simply mimic the move of running, bringing your knee in toward your chest. Make sure to keep your back straight while alternating legs. Do this for 30 seconds.

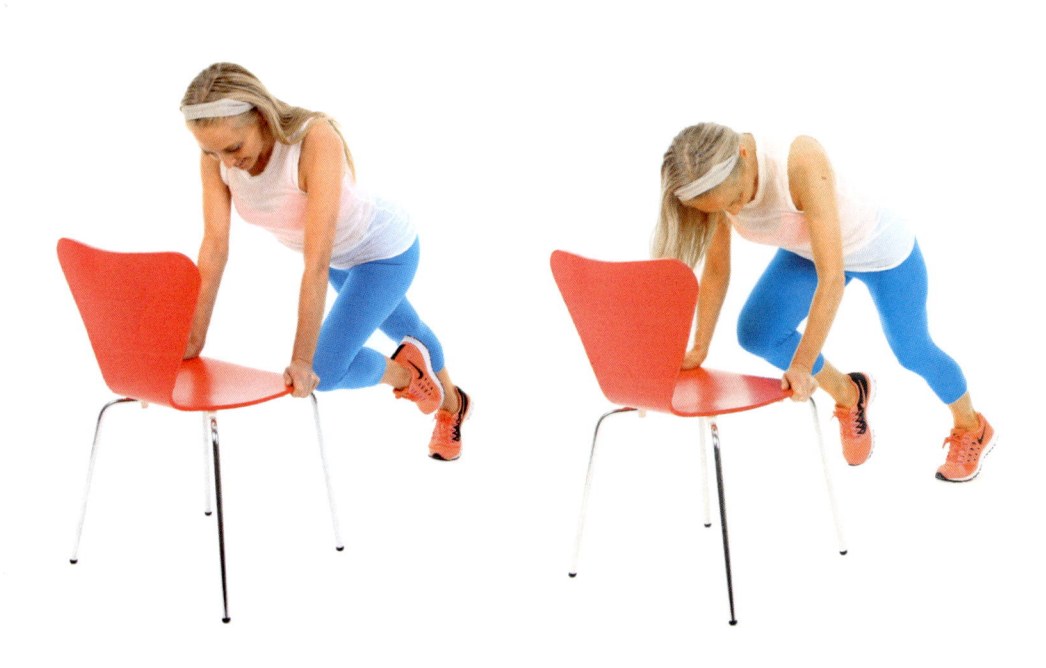

PART II | THE WORKOUTS

EXERCISE 3: CHAIR SQUAT

Face your chair, standing with good posture. Slowly lower into a deep squat, aiming to place your hands on the chair. Hold for a second, and then slowly push back up to the start position. Do 30 repetitions.

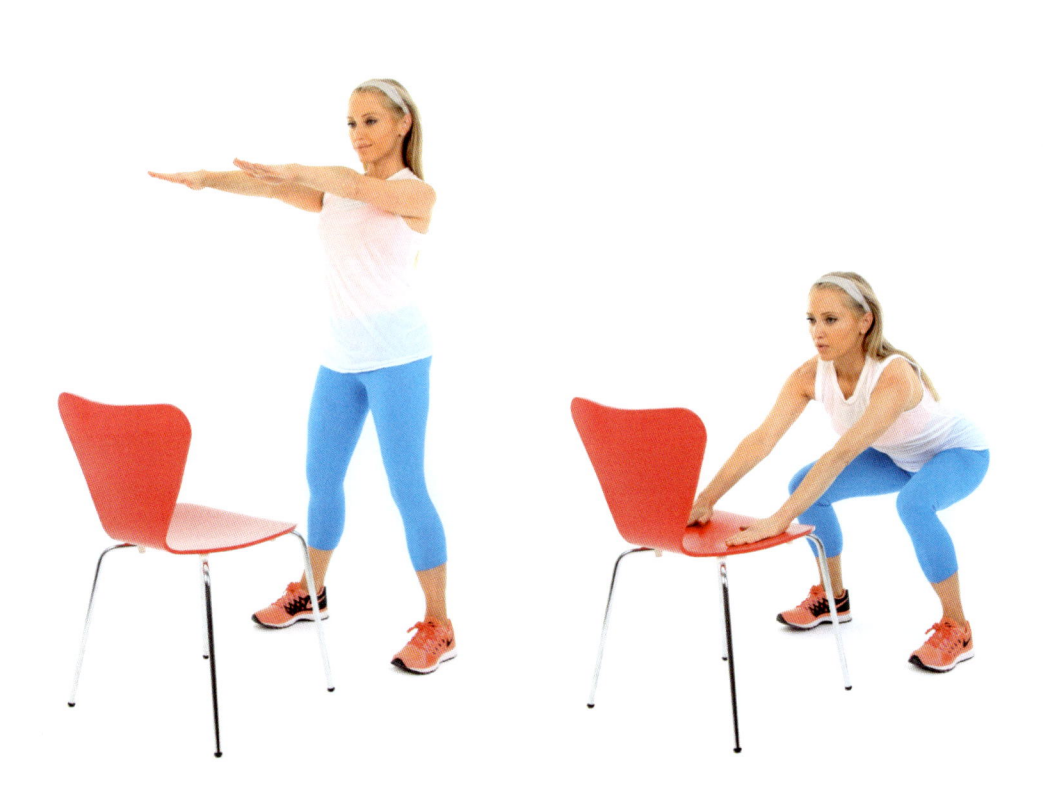

HIIT—HIGH-INTENSITY INTERVAL TRAINING

EXERCISE 4: AB AND ARM TONER

Lean into your chair, after ensuring it is firmly in place and will not slip. Make sure your body is in a straight line, hips dropped, and tummy muscles pulled in. Slowly remove one hand from the chair and touch the opposite shoulder, hold, and then lower the hand. Then lift the opposite hand to touch the other shoulder, always keeping those tummy muscles pulled in. Do 30 repetitions in total.

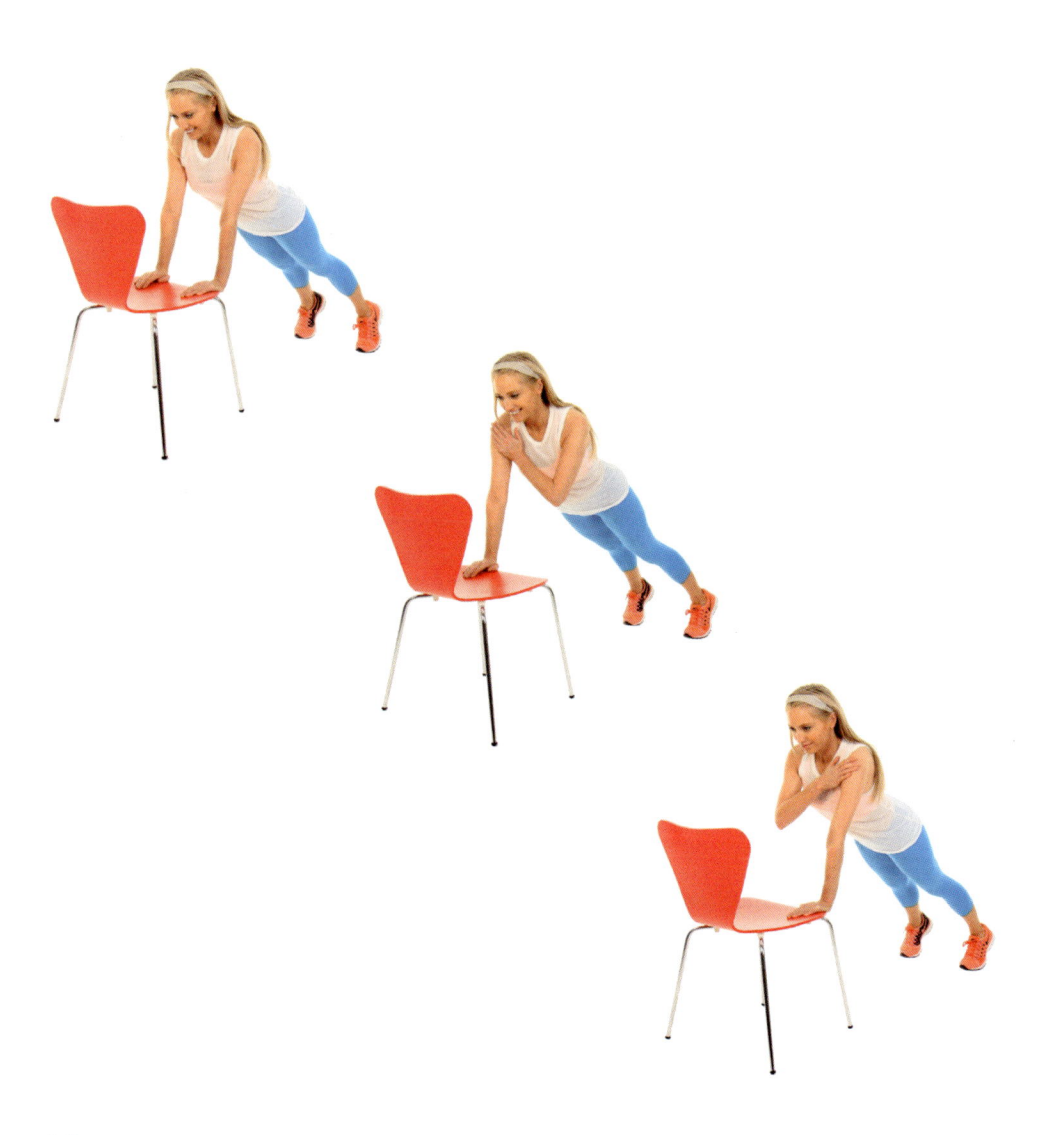

PART II | THE WORKOUTS

EXERCISE 5: ULTIMATE THIGH TONER

Standing side on to your chair, place one leg on the chair and then come into a squat position, making sure you do not let the line of the knee come over your toes. Then squat a little lower, hold for a second, and then come back up. Do 20 repetitions on one leg before changing sides to work the opposite leg.

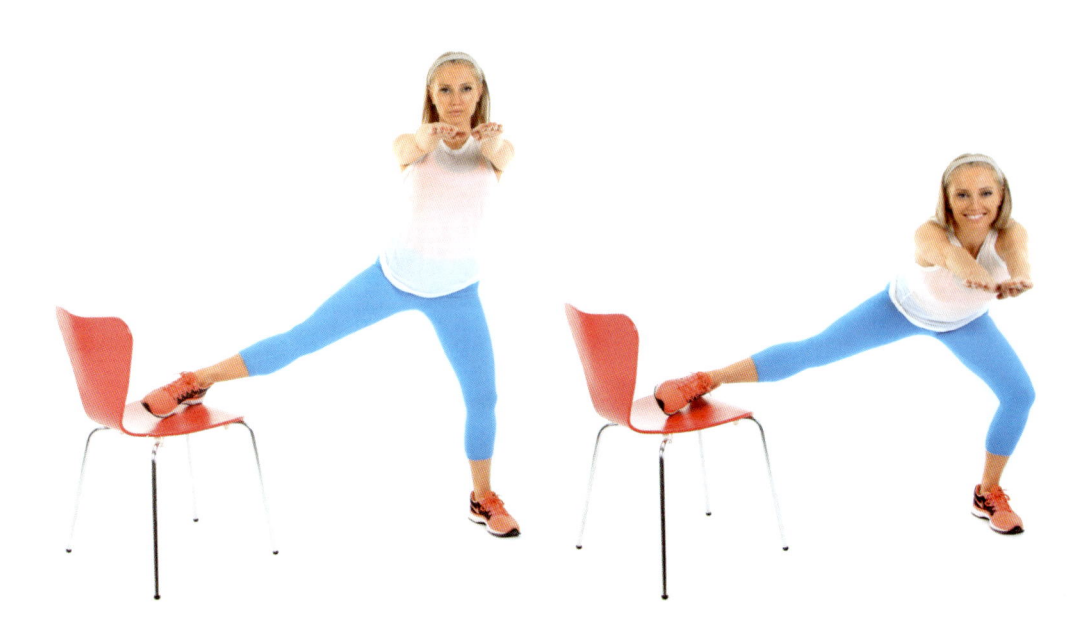

EXERCISE 6: CHAIR AB BLAST

Lie supine with both feet and lower legs resting on the chair. Try to reach up and, with both hands, touch the top of the chair. Hold for a second before lowering. Then try to touch one side of the chair with both hands, then lower, then come back up and touch the center, then lower, and now this time reach around to the opposite side of the chair. Do 40 repetitions. Constantly keep those tummy muscles pulled in.

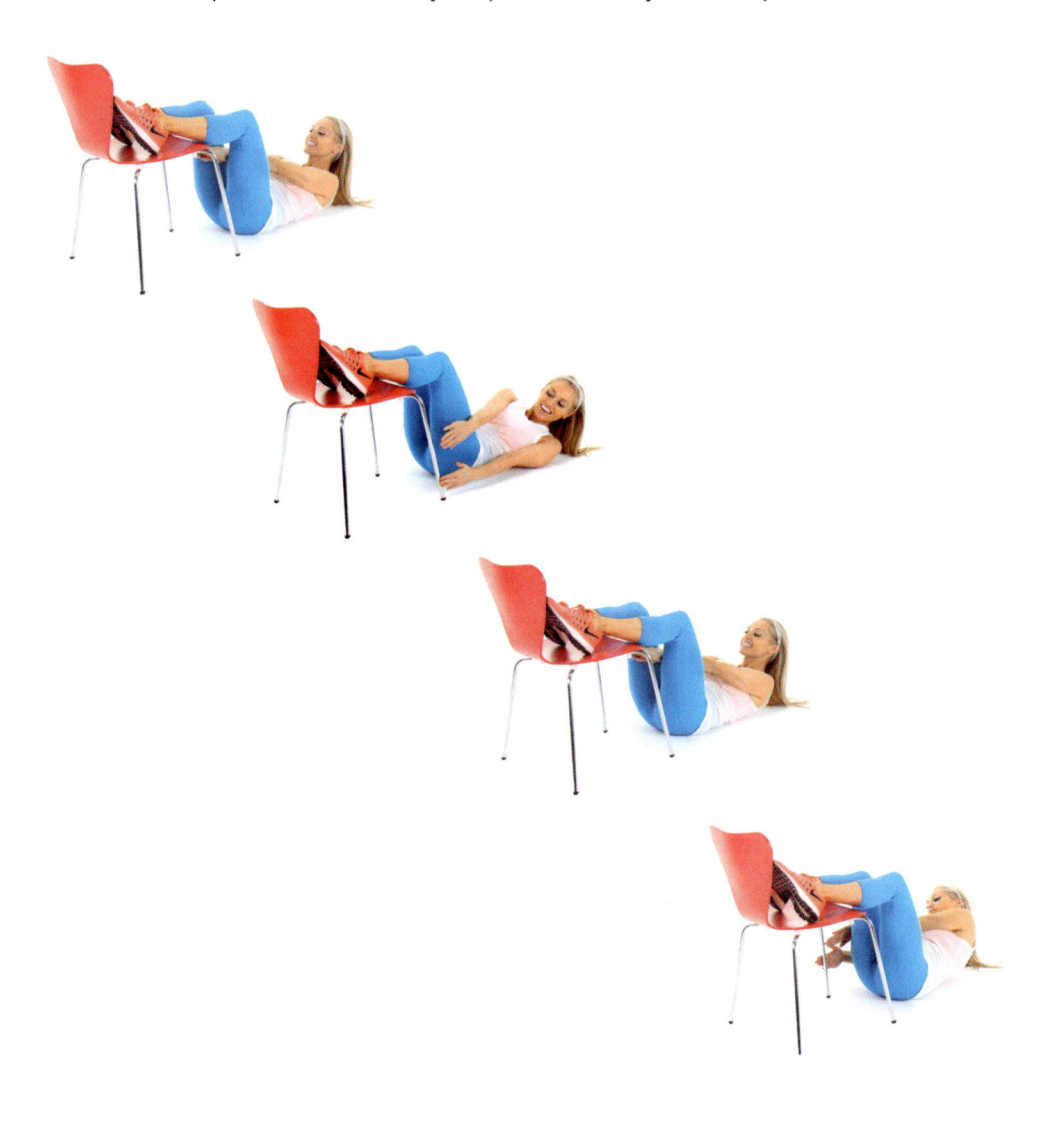

PART II | THE WORKOUTS

EXERCISE 7: CHAIR LUNGE

Step away from your chair and rest one foot on the chair. Extend your arms out in front of you, making sure the front foot is far enough forward that when you lunge down your knee does not go over the line of the toes. Keep your tummy muscles pulled in and upper body straight. Slowly lower yourself to the ground slightly, hold for a second, and then push back up. Do this for 30 seconds on one leg before changing to the other leg.

Once you have completed this workout, make sure you complete your cool-down stretches on pages 35-41.

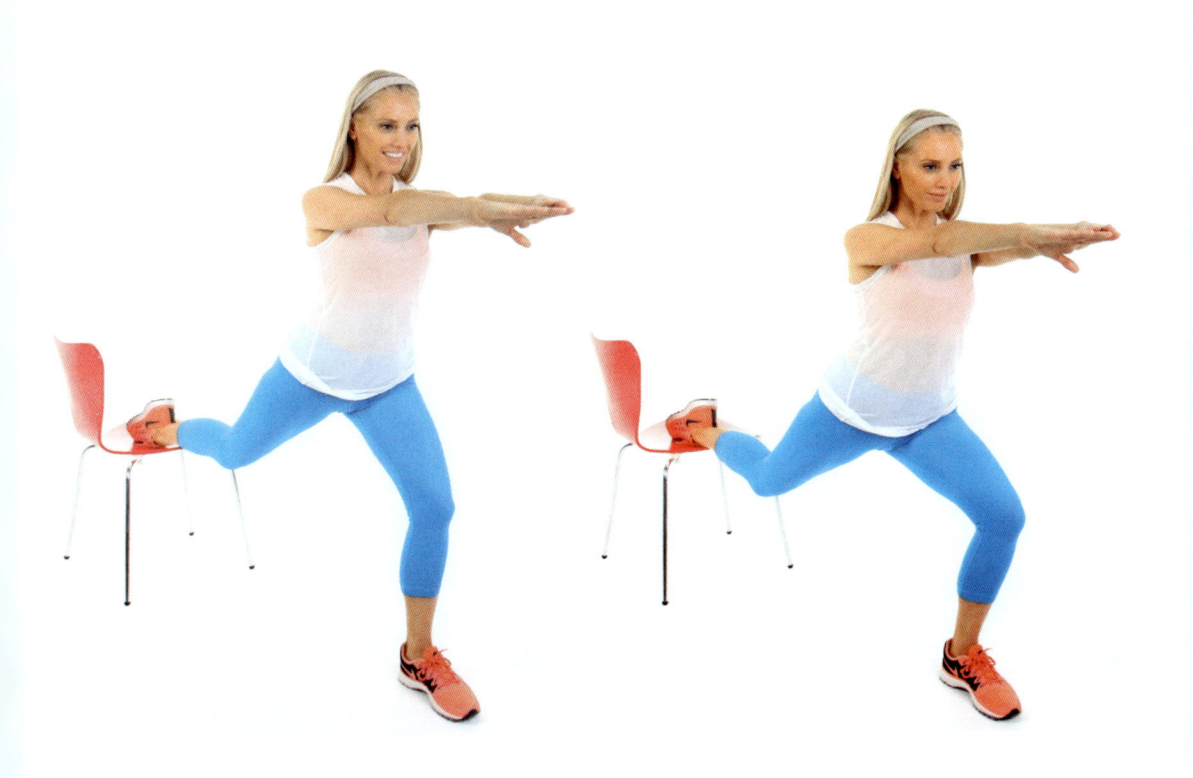

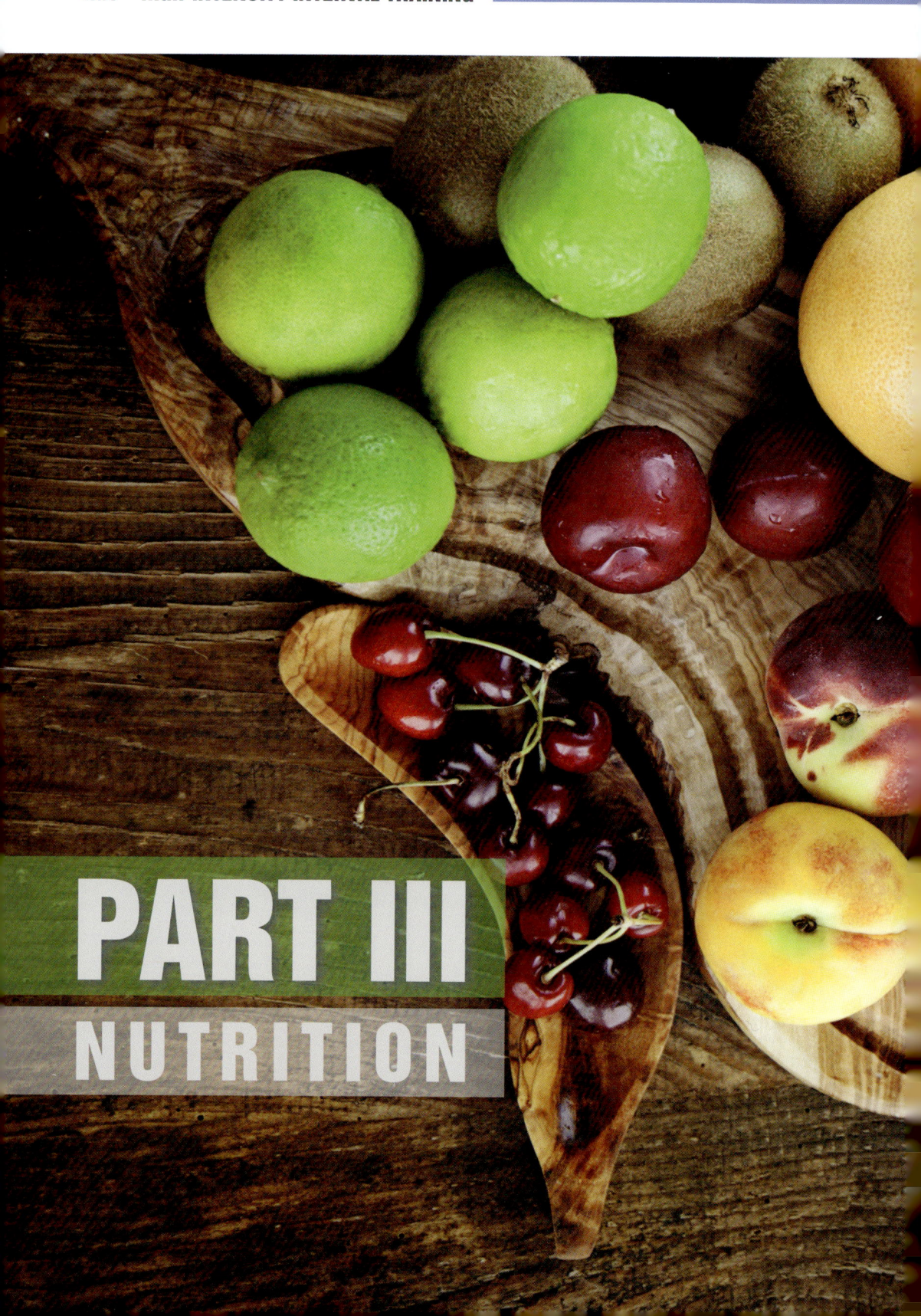

HIIT—HIGH-INTENSITY INTERVAL TRAINING

PART III
NUTRITION

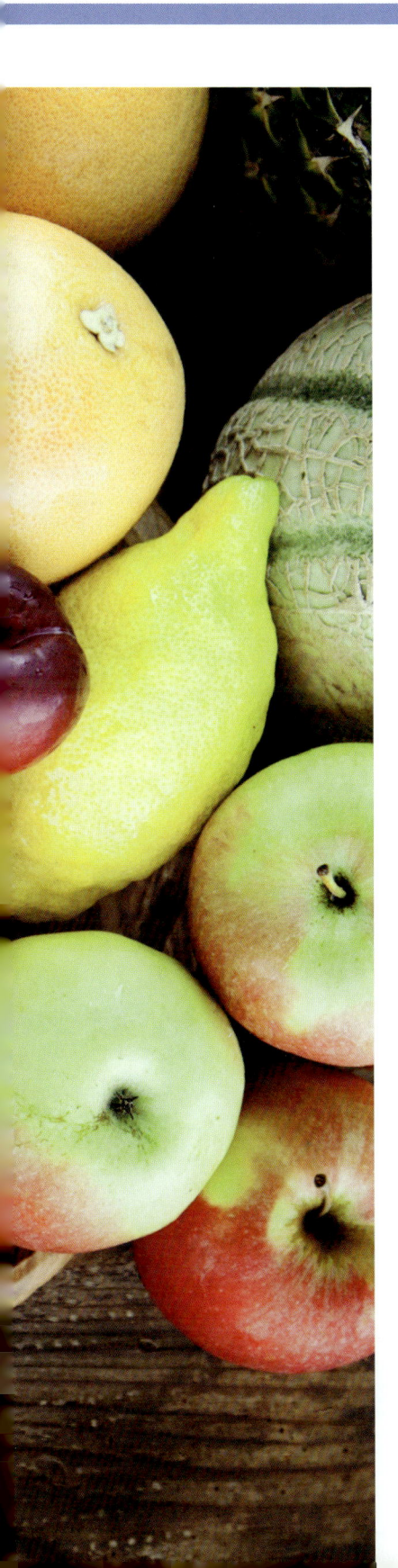

26 LEARN ABOUT CLEAN FIT FOOD

Get faster results from your HIIT workouts with the right nutrition.

To get truly amazing results with my HIIT workouts, we need to combine them with what I call clean fit food, so welcome to my Fit Kitchen. I am going to show you how easy it is to eat healthy and super tasty food with no weighing scales. We are using clean, natural foods with some unique but, trust me, delicious combinations. I and all my friends and family have tried and tested these (many times, as they are that delicious). You saw these meals and snack ideas here first, and this is my 7-Day HIIT FIT Food.

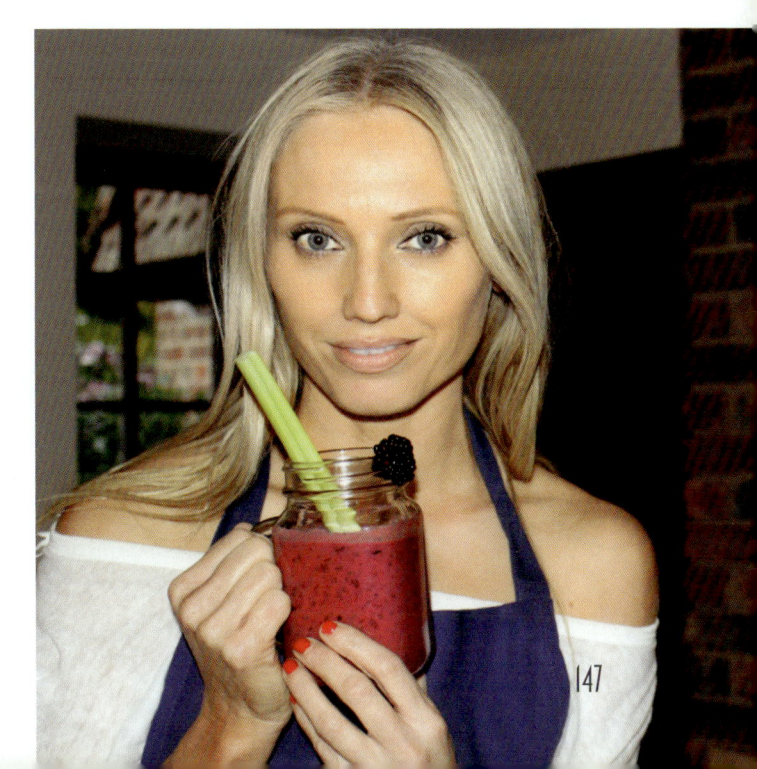

HIIT—HIGH-INTENSITY INTERVAL TRAINING

As with anything in life, knowledge is power, so I want to break down the basics of nutrition, because I believe the more we understand how our body works and what it needs, the easier it is to stick to healthy living.

The most important thing to remember with your diet is that this is the fuel you give your body, and we want to focus on feeding it the healthiest and best quality fuel there is by eating clean fit foods (and by this, I mean unprocessed). This really makes sense when you think about it. If you want to feel in optimal health and look and feel your best and have plenty of energy throughout the day, then you can have all this by simply ensuring every mouthful is good quality.

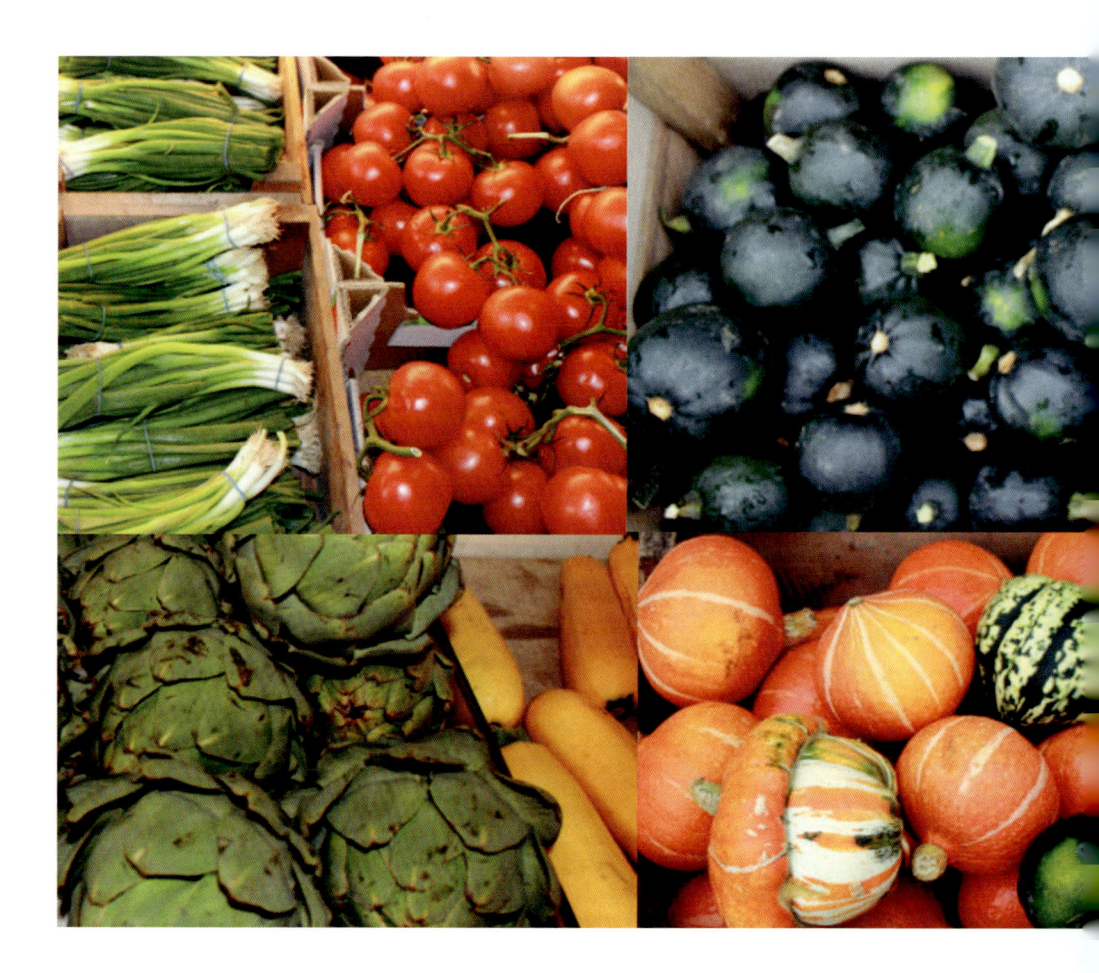

27 WHAT MAKES A HEALTHY CLEAN FIT DIET

A healthy diet should consist of a wide variety of foods. This way you ensure your body is getting all the nutrients it needs. Many fad diets restrict us from eating certain food groups, but the fact is that eating a healthy well-balanced diet can be easy and tasty.

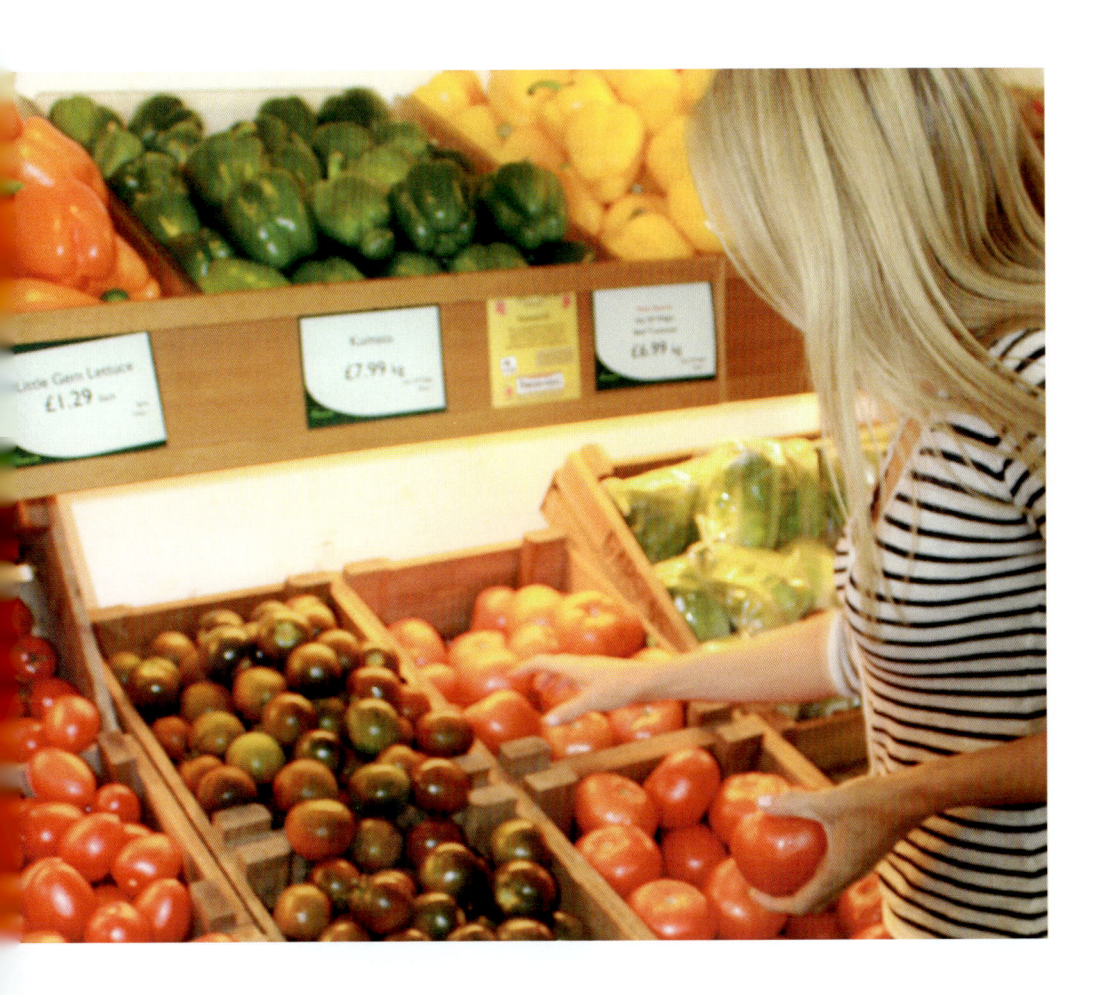

YOUR BODY NEEDS ALL THESE COMPONENTS OF NUTRITION:

Carbohydrates: So many people think these are bad and cut them out of their diet, but we need these daily to give us energy.

Protein: This is needed to help the body repair itself and build tissue.

Fats: (Yes, again, these are good, as long as it is good fat.) These help supply longterm energy so that the body is fully charged.

Fiber: It is essential to help maintain good digestive health.

Minerals: These are needed to help control metabolism and cellular activity.

Vitamins: These simply help make the body work properly.

If you daily eat all these food components, you will feel in optimal health. But if you deprive your body of these nutrients, you won't function properly! It's as simple as that!

Here is an example shopping list that contains all the right food choices that will look after you and your health.

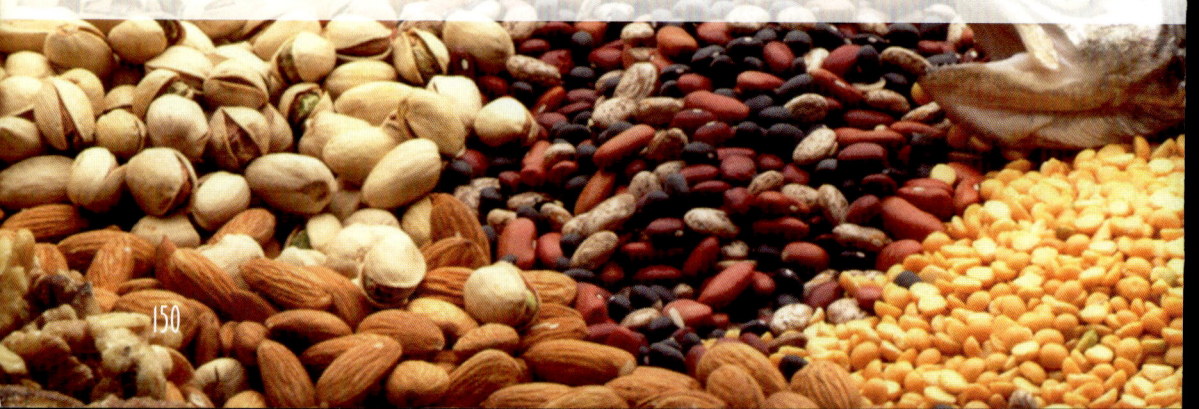

Shopping List:

Oats, couscous,
Whole-grain pasta and rice
Rye bread, whole-grain pitas
Chicken breasts
Salmon and cod fillets
Turkey
Lean beef
Tuna or sardines
Ham and turkey slices
Frozen prawns
Lentils
Kidney beans
Chickpeas
Peas
Fruits and Vegetables:
- apples, bananas, melon, dates, oranges, blueberries,
- kiwi, grapes, grapefruit
- sweet potatoes, spinach, celery
- salad leaves, herbs
- avocados, beetroot, peppers
- radish, courgettes, onion
- mushrooms

Nuts and raisins
Dried coconut
Honey
Mustard
Seeds
Eggs, milk
Low-fat natural youghurt
Cottage cheese, mozarella

HIIT—HIGH-INTENSITY INTERVAL TRAINING

28 THE DANGERS OF SUGAR

Sugar is one of the biggest causes of obesity and serious health conditions! This white stuff can be a highly addictive drug that many of us have become hooked on without even realizing it, and this substance is hidden in all sorts of foods, sauces, and drinks! You may think you don't have much sugar in your diet, but here is an example of a client of mine, Jemma, who was struggling to shift those last few pounds. She was convinced that she did not have much sugar in her diet.

She never sprinkled it on her cereal and always had tea without sugar. She just had one coffee a day, but this is where she was an addict without realizing it!

This is taken from Jemma's food diary, and I have bolded everything with sugar in it.

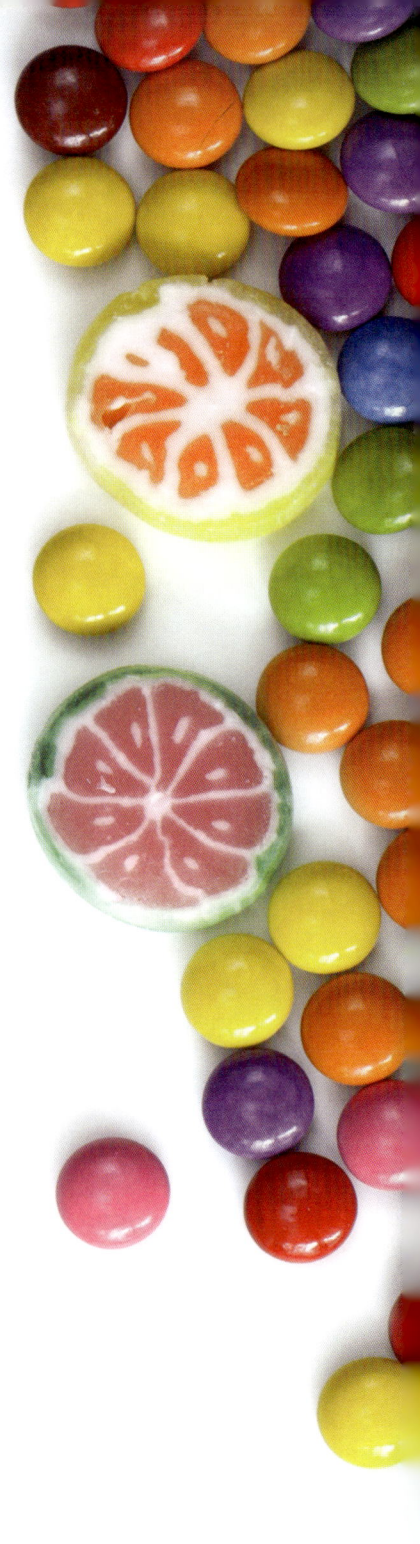

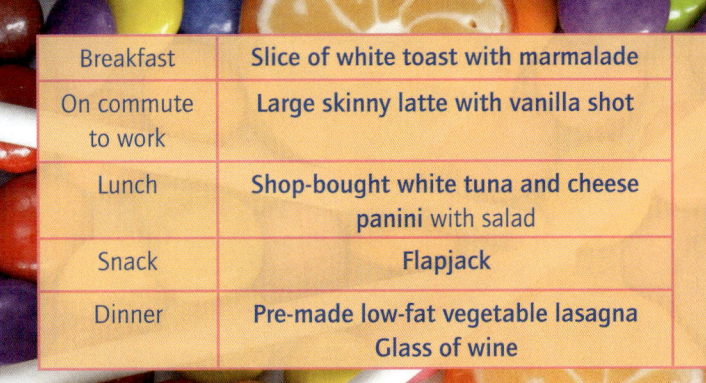

Breakfast	**Slice of white toast with marmalade**
On commute to work	**Large skinny latte with vanilla shot**
Lunch	**Shop-bought white tuna and cheese panini** with salad
Snack	**Flapjack**
Dinner	**Pre-made low-fat vegetable lasagna Glass of wine**

Even though Jemma was not eating anything deep-fried or eating chips, cookies, doughnuts, or soda, she was still consuming vast amounts of sugar. No wonder she complained of bloating and feeling tired.

Refined sugar is found in most processed foods, and this is why we need to go back to eating a healthy unprocessed diet. Beware of clever packaging labels on foods that tell us they are good for us yet often have hidden sugar!

I gave Jemma a Fit Food Diet for her to try which was similar to hers, but with no REFINED sugar.

Breakfast	1 slice of whole-grain toast topped with a thin layer of cottage cheese and sliced strawberries
On commute to work	Medium soy latte with no vanilla shot
Lunch	Rocket and tuna salad with kidney and lima beans
Snack	Homemade vanilla popcorn
Dinner	Grilled vegetables with chicken breast and sweet potato mash

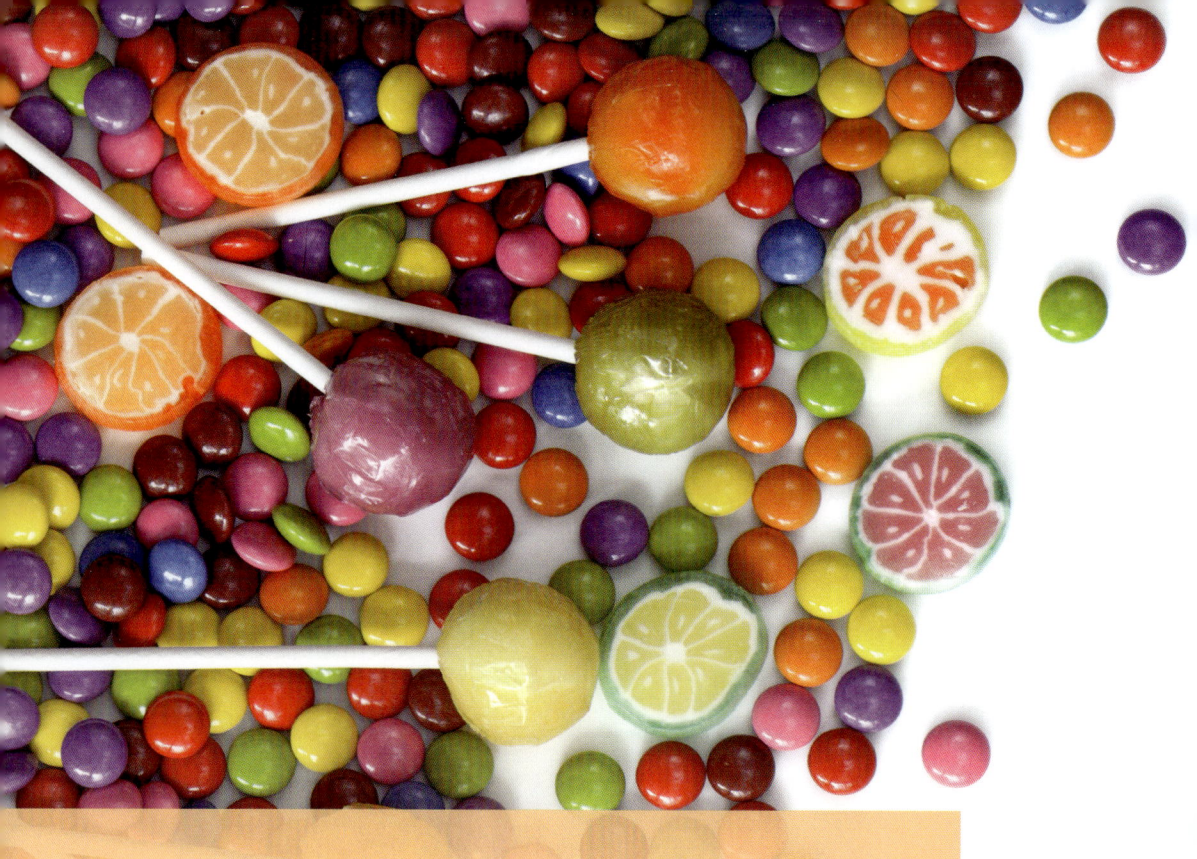

This day's diet had no refined sugar, and Jemma said for once she was not bloated and felt full and satisfied after each meal and had plenty of energy.

The problem is that nowadays sugar is in everything. When I was a child, sugar would just be associated with having that cake or cookie, but since the food manufacturers started putting extra white stuff in all sorts of foods, especially things like cereals, breads, drinks, and worse, kids' foods, it is now being consumed so much more. This is one of the biggest reasons for the rise in obesity.

But if we simply eat clean fit food we can ensure that the refined white sugars stay well out of our diet, which then means we keep that healthy body weight, reduce the risk of disease, and wake up every morning feeling great.

29 SIZE MATTERS!

Nowadays foods portions are way too big and have doubled and even tripled in size. The dinner plate, which 20 years ago on average was 9 inches, has now doubled to 18 inches, so no wonder we are all getting bigger, as we are simply consuming too many calories. So know what size portions you should be eating. This is a simple tool to familiarize yourself with. And this guide of mine will help keep you on track, as size really does matter.

- Vegetables: small saucepan
- Lean meats: size of a deck of playing cards
- Pastas, pulses, grains, cereal: size of a tennis ball
- Cheese or dairy products: size of a matchbox
- Fruit: size of a tea cup
- Fish: size of a checkbook
- Oils, honey, and dressings: size of thimble

30 THE CLEAN FIT FOOD SCALE

So let's start eating fit food and enjoying every mouthful, and better still feeling great after we have eaten it.

TIP: Make it a rule of thumb now that every time you eat, you quickly assess the standard of your food choice by using this scale of mine. And allow yourself a good few minutes to think if you really need to eat the food that is in the scale 3 bracket. Sometimes we crave the wrong foods when we are tired, so perhaps even something as simple as a quick 5-minute walk around the block before you eat that chocolate bar may help supercharge those energy levels. Then you might realize it was the exercise you needed, not the chocolate!

The Scale	The Food Choice	How You Feel After Eating
1	Natural and clean, no added, processed, or artificial ingredients	Great and full of energy
2	50/50: half natural and half artificial	Tired
3	Completely processed and with artificial ingredients	Tired, bloated, and lethargic

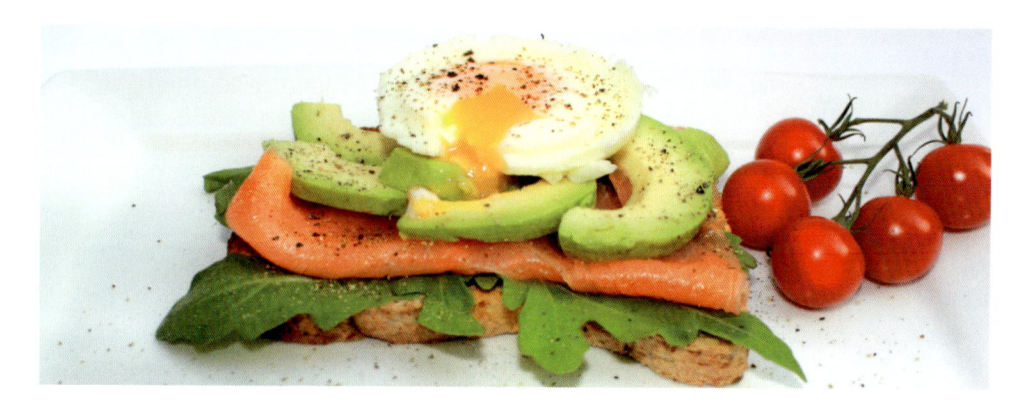

Sunday Brunch

This delicious meal will definitely score a 1.

PART III | NUTRITION

31 MY 7-DAY CLEAN FIT FOOD EATING PLAN

Food should taste good and, more importantly, be a great source of all your vitamins and minerals.

Food does more than stop you feeling hungry—it also helps provide you with energy. The better quality food you eat, the more you give to your body. A great saying I heard once was "every bite we take will either heal our body or destroy our body."

It does get you thinking! So one of the best ways to eat is to stick to the rule: 80 percent of the time stick to the good stuff, then you are allowed 20 percent of the not-so-good stuff if you are tempted to eat the less tasty and crave the premade choice, but I hope with this book you will see how delicious these clean fit foods are that these will be all you crave.

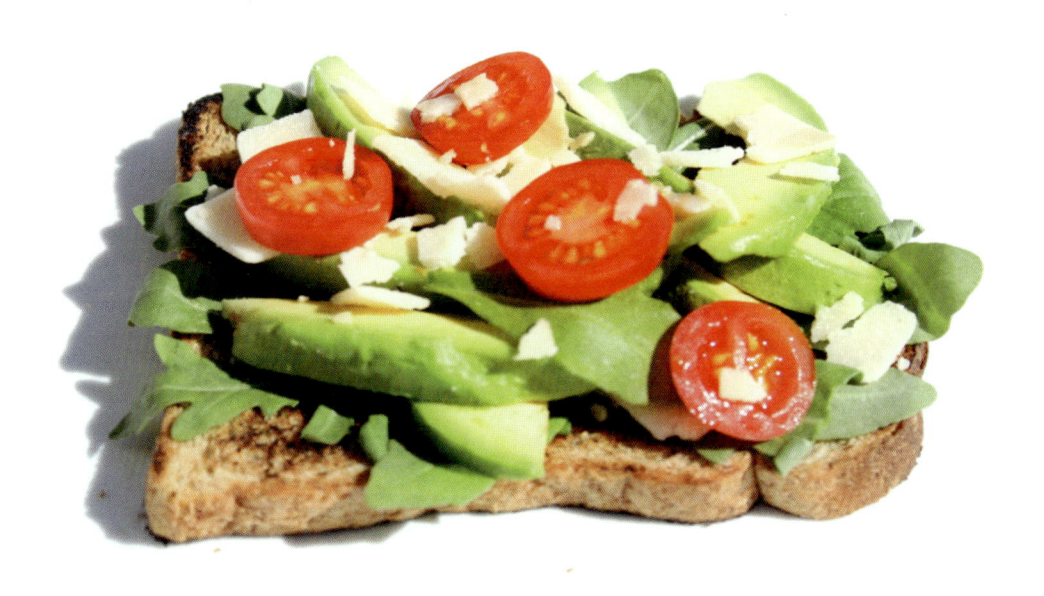

Open Sandwich

HIIT—HIGH INTENSITY INTERVAL TRAINING

DAY 1

BREAKFAST

Oats and raspberry breakfast pudding

Add some oats, then a splash of low-fat natural yogurt. Add chopped banana and raspberries. You can sprinkle on a few extra seeds and dried fruit to give it that extra crunch.

SNACK

Small pieces of cheese with an apple

LUNCH

Whole-grain pita with salad and hummus

SNACK

Oatcake topped with half of an avocado

DINNER

Stir-fried beef with garlic served on brown rice with peas

PART III | NUTRITION

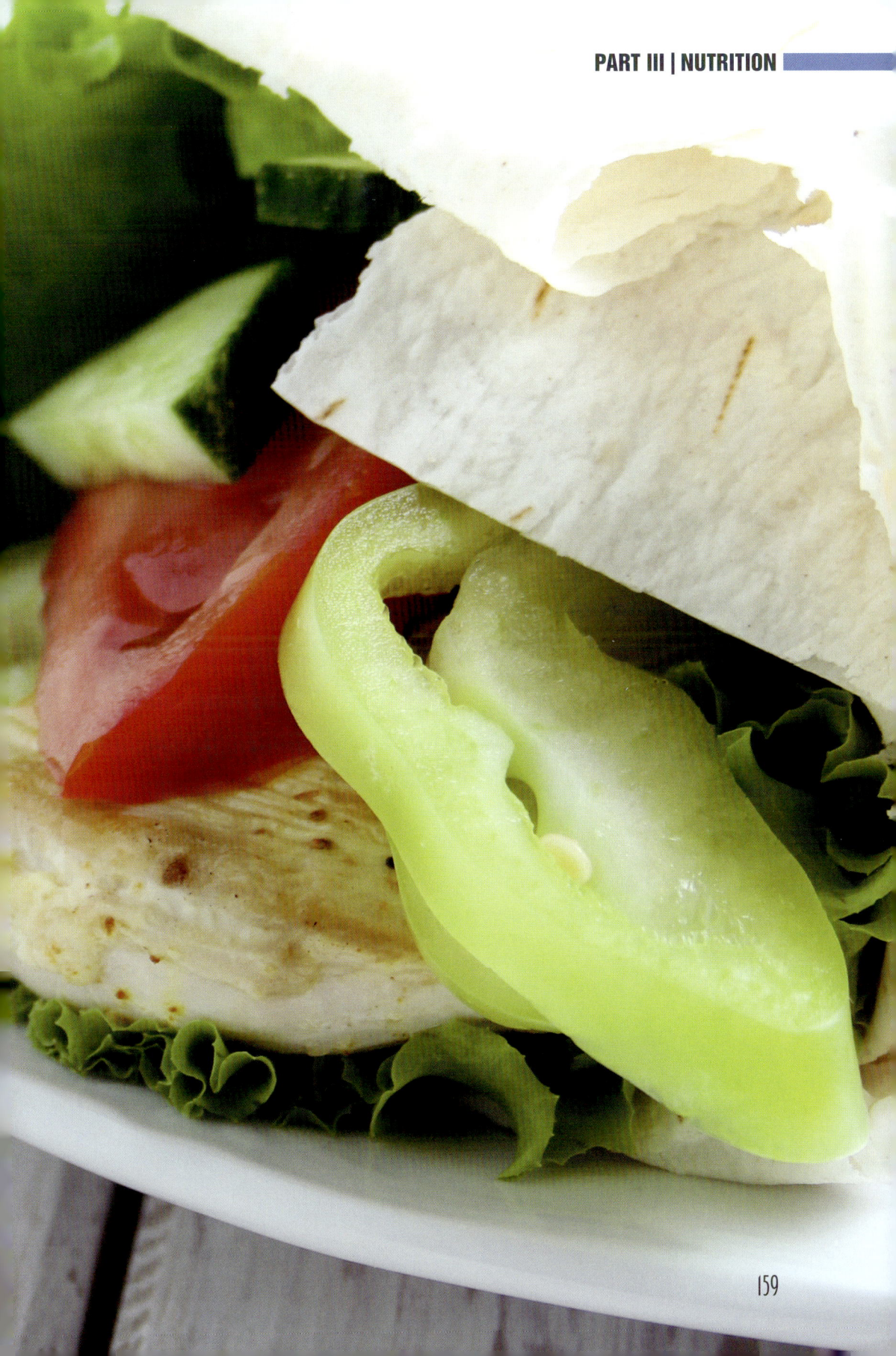

HIIT—HIGH INTENSITY INTERVAL TRAINING

DAY 2

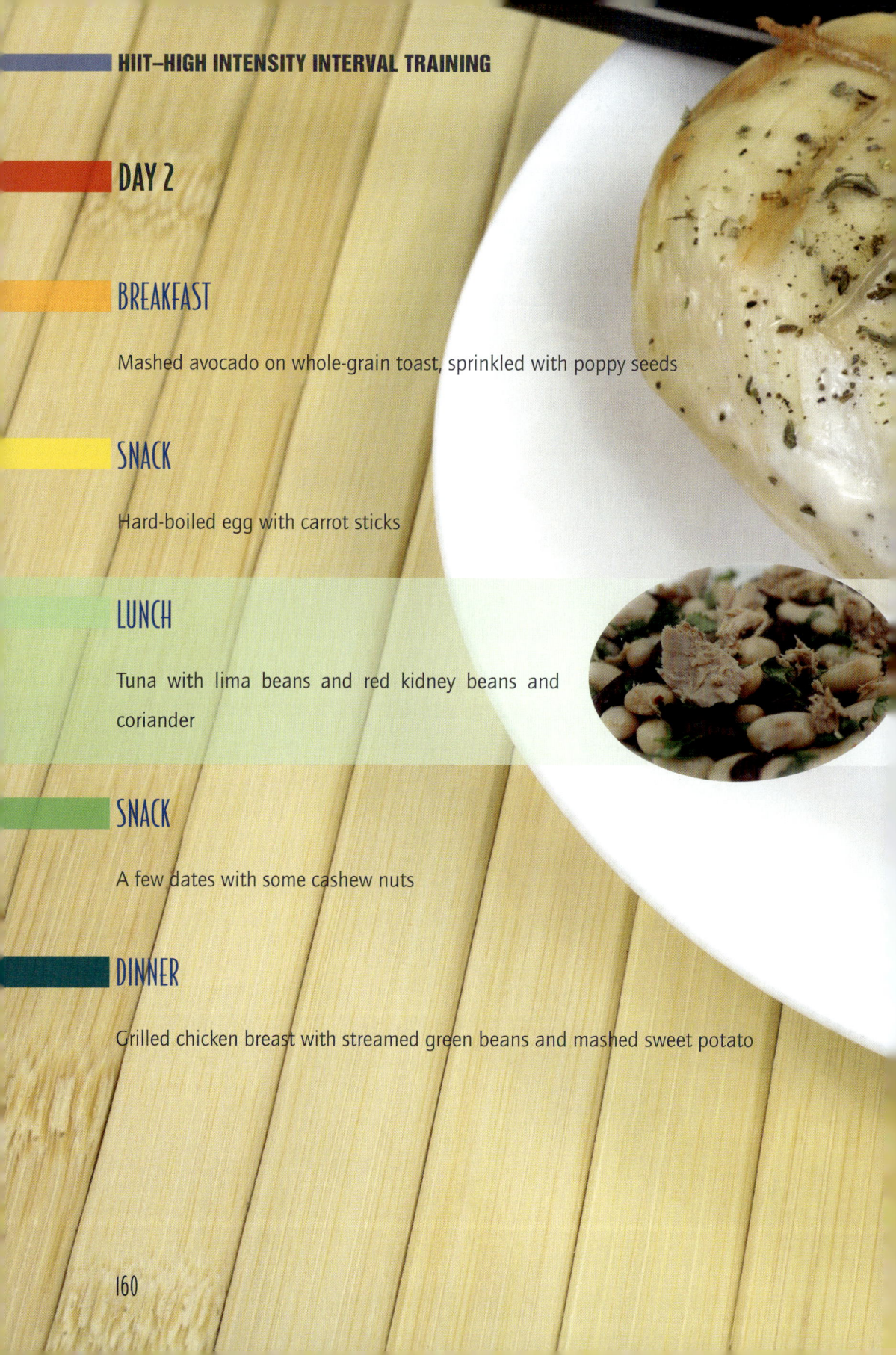

BREAKFAST

Mashed avocado on whole-grain toast, sprinkled with poppy seeds

SNACK

Hard-boiled egg with carrot sticks

LUNCH

Tuna with lima beans and red kidney beans and coriander

SNACK

A few dates with some cashew nuts

DINNER

Grilled chicken breast with streamed green beans and mashed sweet potato

PART III | NUTRITION

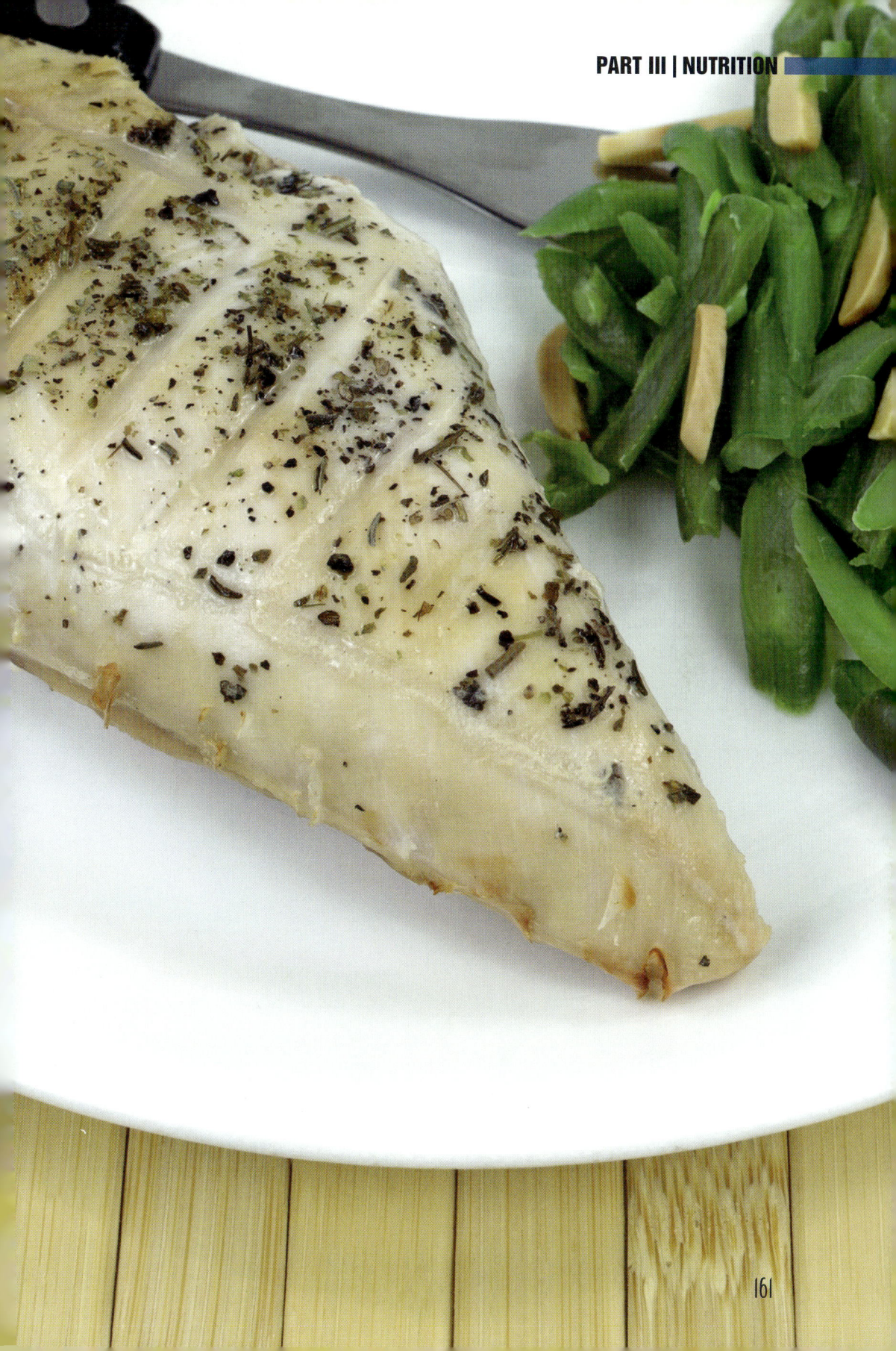

HIIT–HIGH INTENSITY INTERVAL TRAINING

DAY 3

BREAKFAST

Bowl of whole-grain cereal topped with some blueberries

SNACK

Super-Green Smoothie
Spinach, apple, celery, pear, and then top with goji berries and chia seeds

LUNCH

Turkey sandwich with grated carrots and hummus

SNACK

Red pepper sticks with cottage cheese as a dip

DINNER

Grilled marinated garlic king prawn kebabs served on lemon-flavored brown rice

PART III | NUTRITION

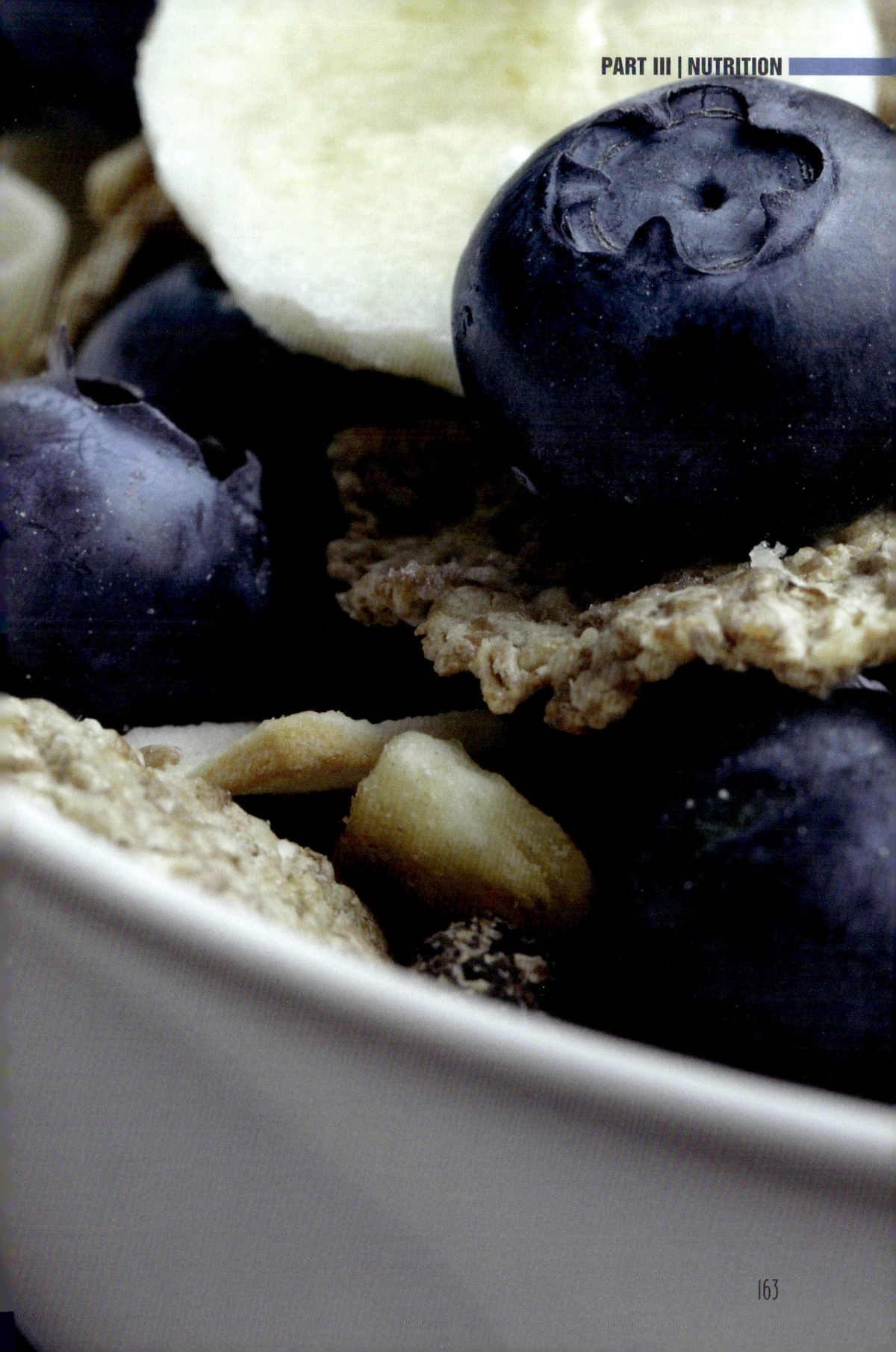

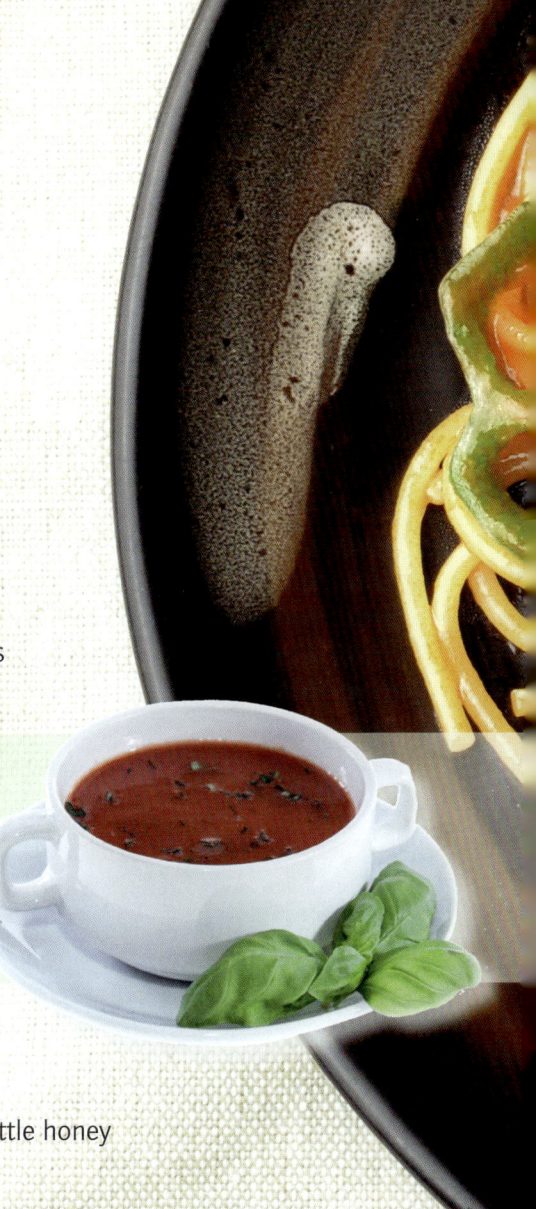

HIIT–HIGH INTENSITY INTERVAL TRAINING

DAY 4

BREAKFAST

Scrambled eggs with grilled field mushrooms

SNACK

A few almonds with a couple of dried apricots

LUNCH

Low-fat tomato soup with half a whole-grain pita

SNACK

Small low-fat yogurt with added oats and a little honey

DINNER

Roasted vegetables served with whole-grain pasta

PART III | NUTRITION

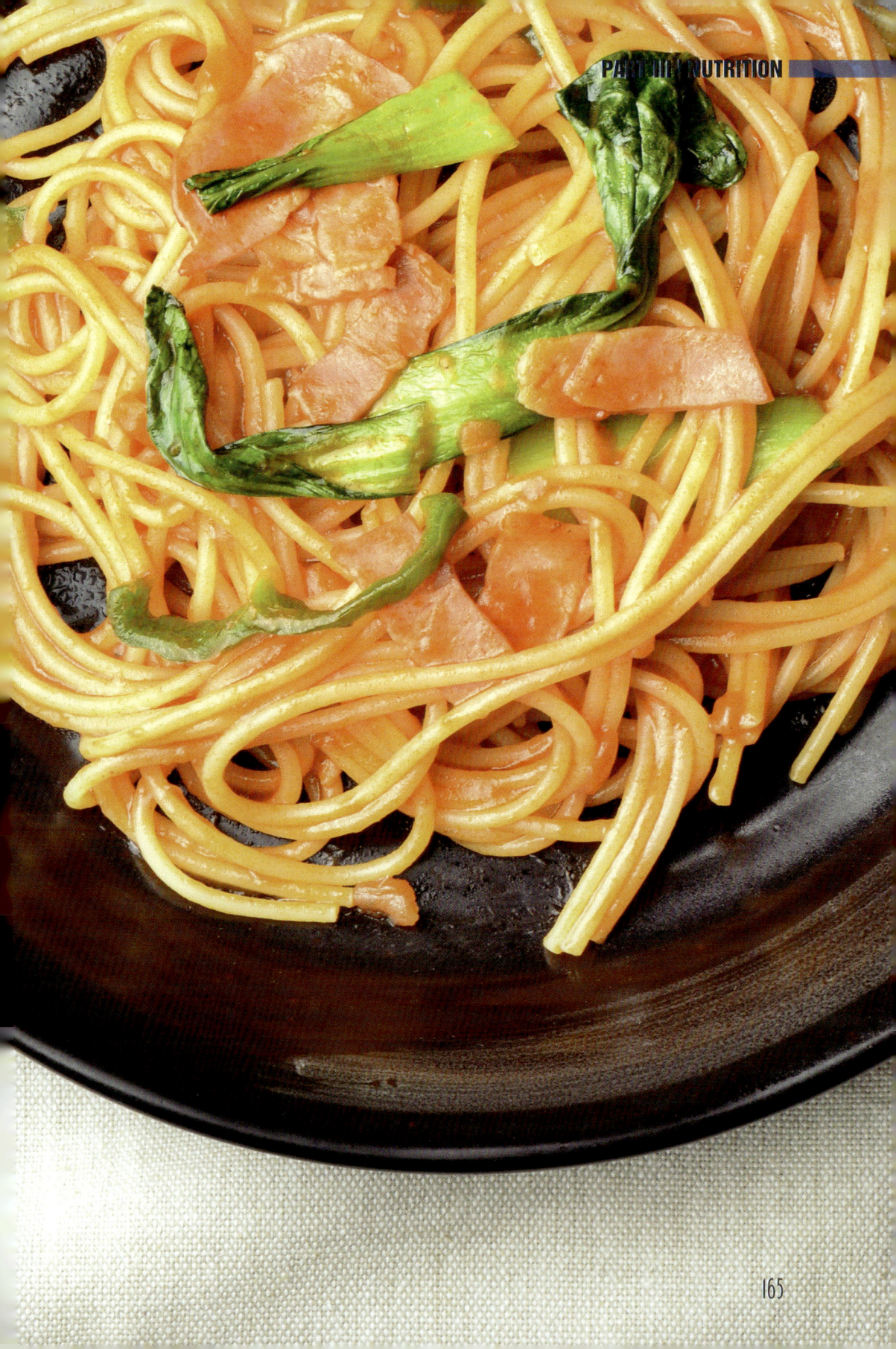

HIIT–HIGH INTENSITY INTERVAL TRAINING

DAY 5

BREAKFAST

Warm oatmeal with pear chunks and a sprinkle of cinnamon

SNACK

Oatcake topped with a banana and a few almond flakes

LUNCH

Avocado with tuna and red pepper and chia seeds

SNACK

Celery stick and low-fat cream cheese

DINNER

Salmon fillet served on quinoa with steamed broccoli

PART III | NUTRITION

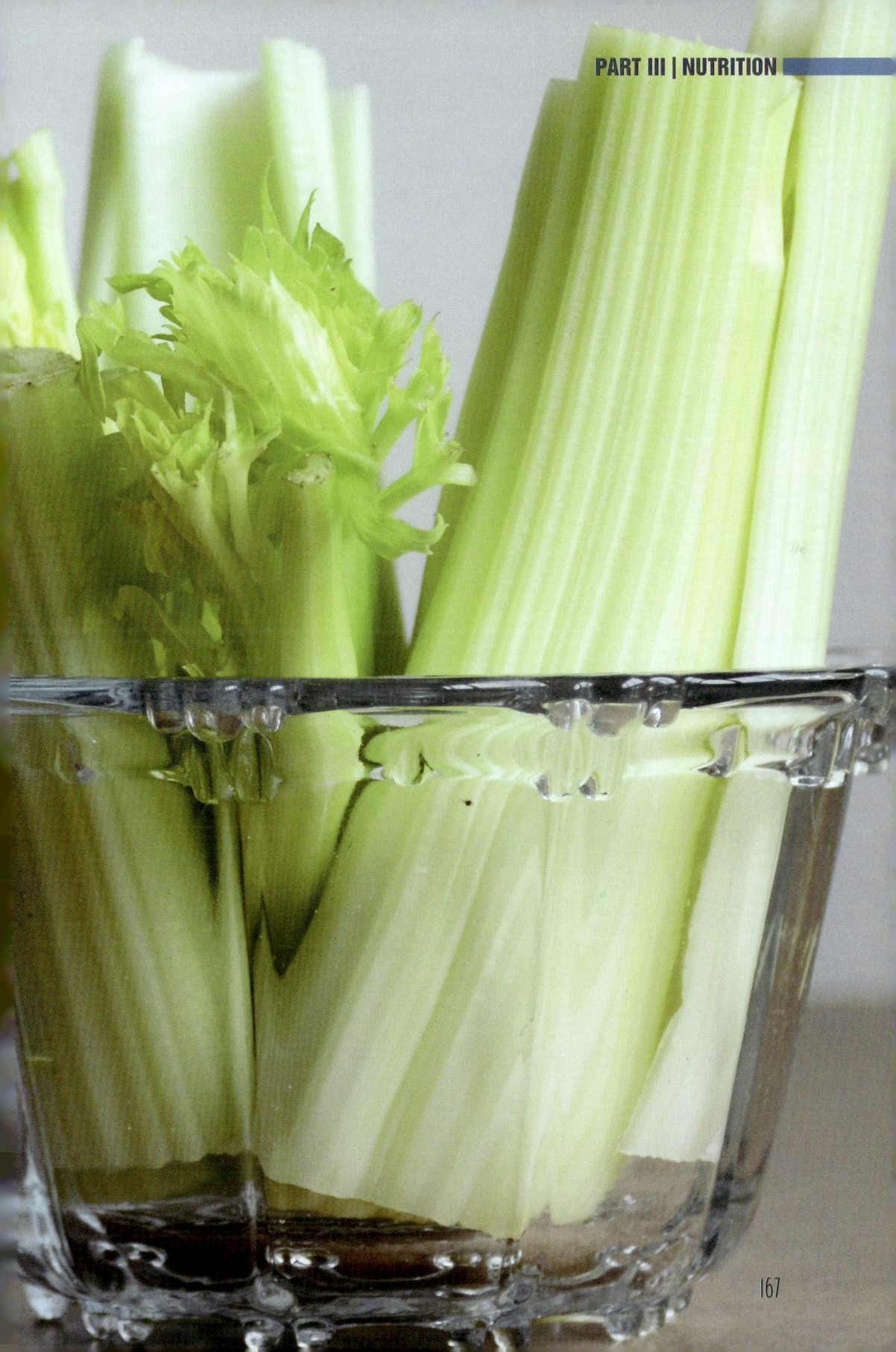

DAY 6

BREAKFAST

Poached egg on toast with half of an avocado

SNACK

Small yogurt with added poppy seeds

LUNCH

Grated courgette with feta cheese and cherry tomatoes, pumpkin, and pine nut salad

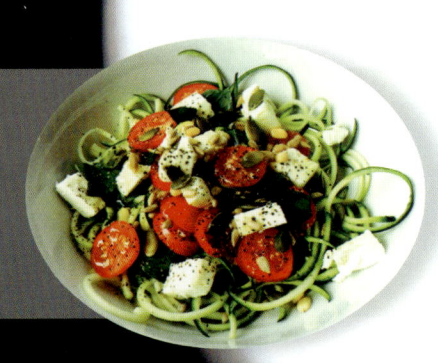

SNACK

Oatcake with half of a mashed avocado

DINNER

Grilled chicken breast with a sweet jacket potato and french green beans

PART III | NUTRITION

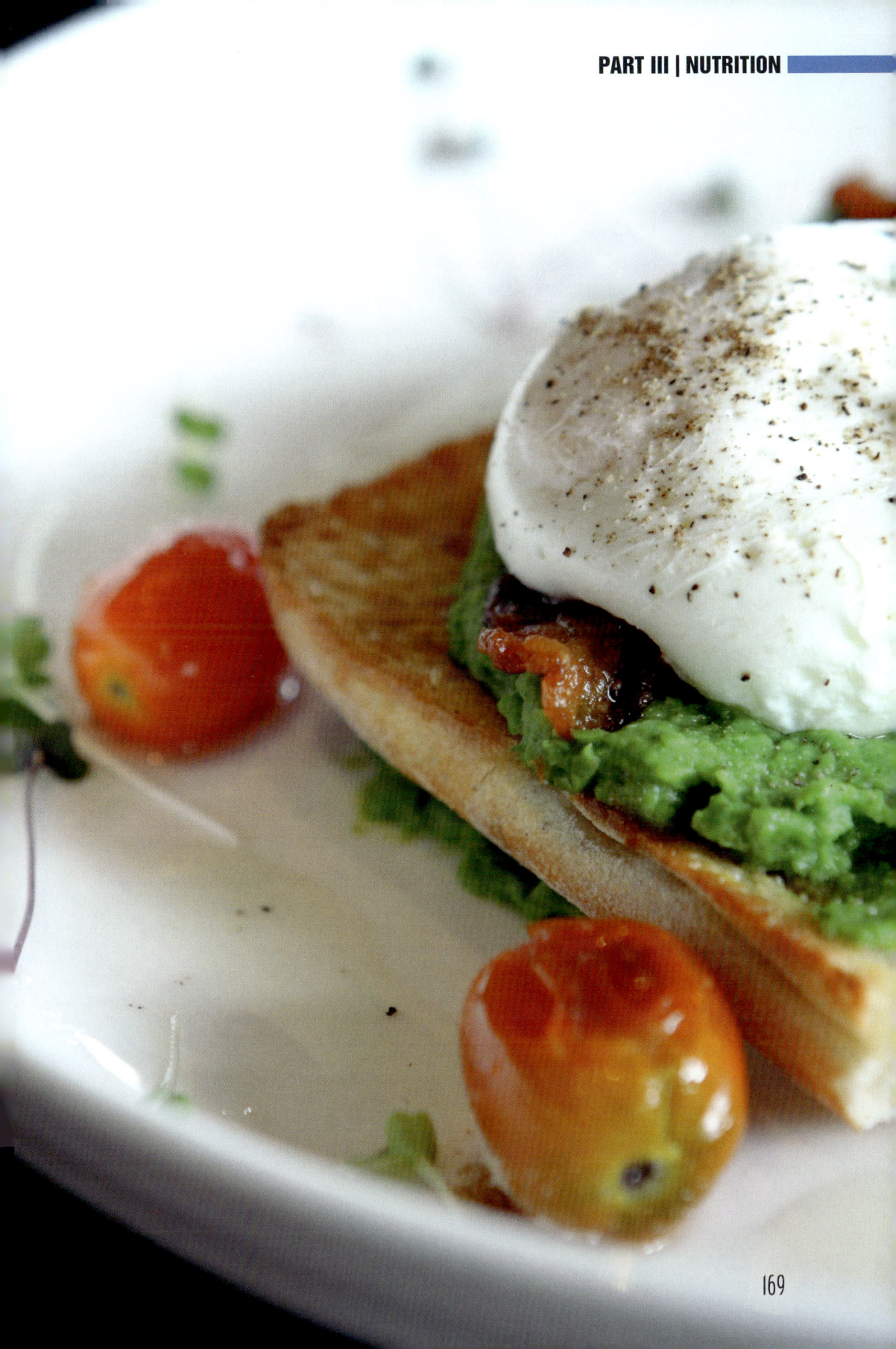

HIIT—HIGH INTENSITY INTERVAL TRAINING

DAY 7

BREAKFAST

Grilled lean bacon with scrambled eggs

SNACK

Hot milk drink with a banana

LUNCH

Whole-grain pita stuffed with rocket, mozzarella, cherry tomatoes, and a few pine nuts

SNACK

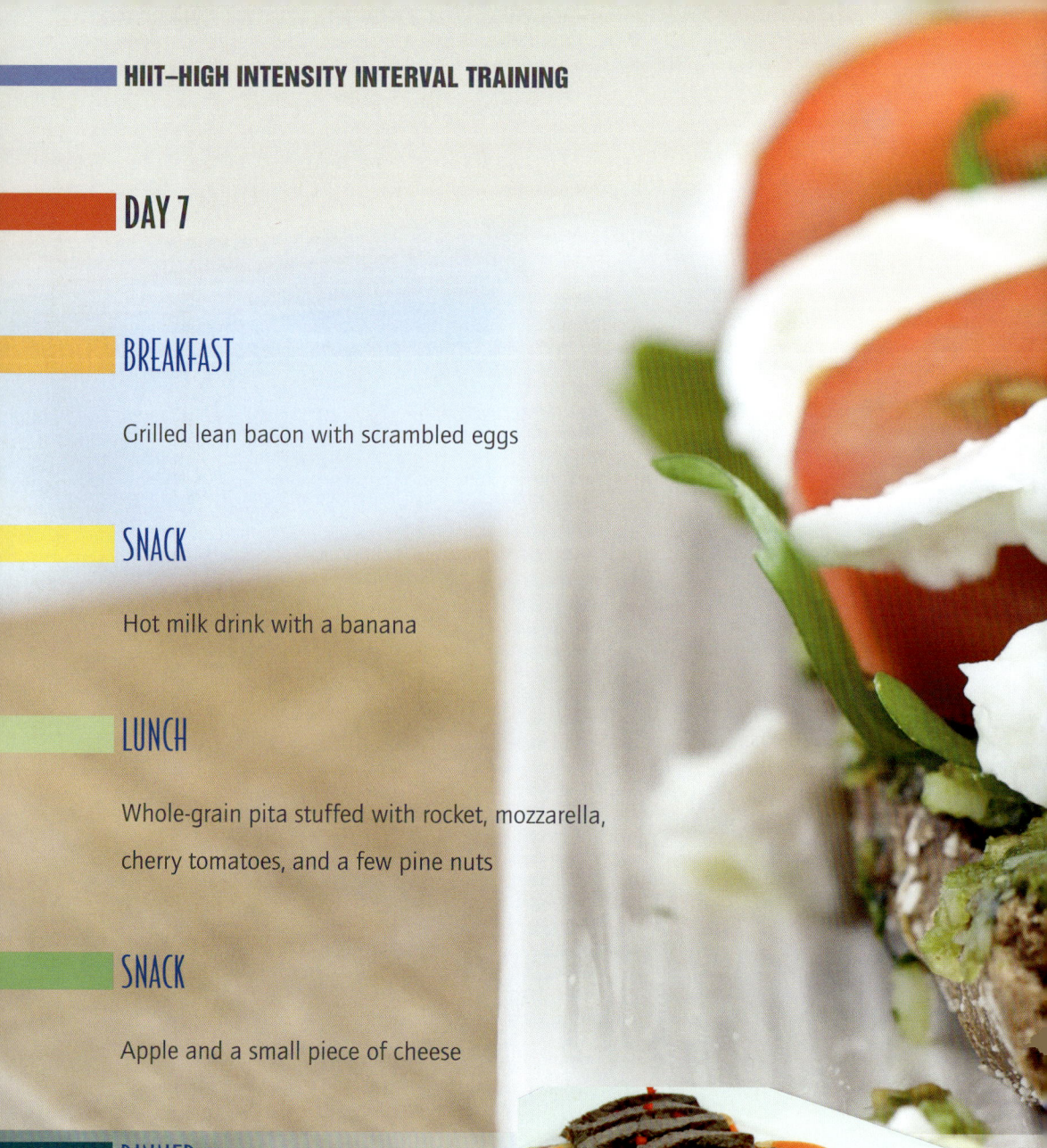

Apple and a small piece of cheese

DINNER

Lean beef vegetable stir fry

PART III | NUTRITION

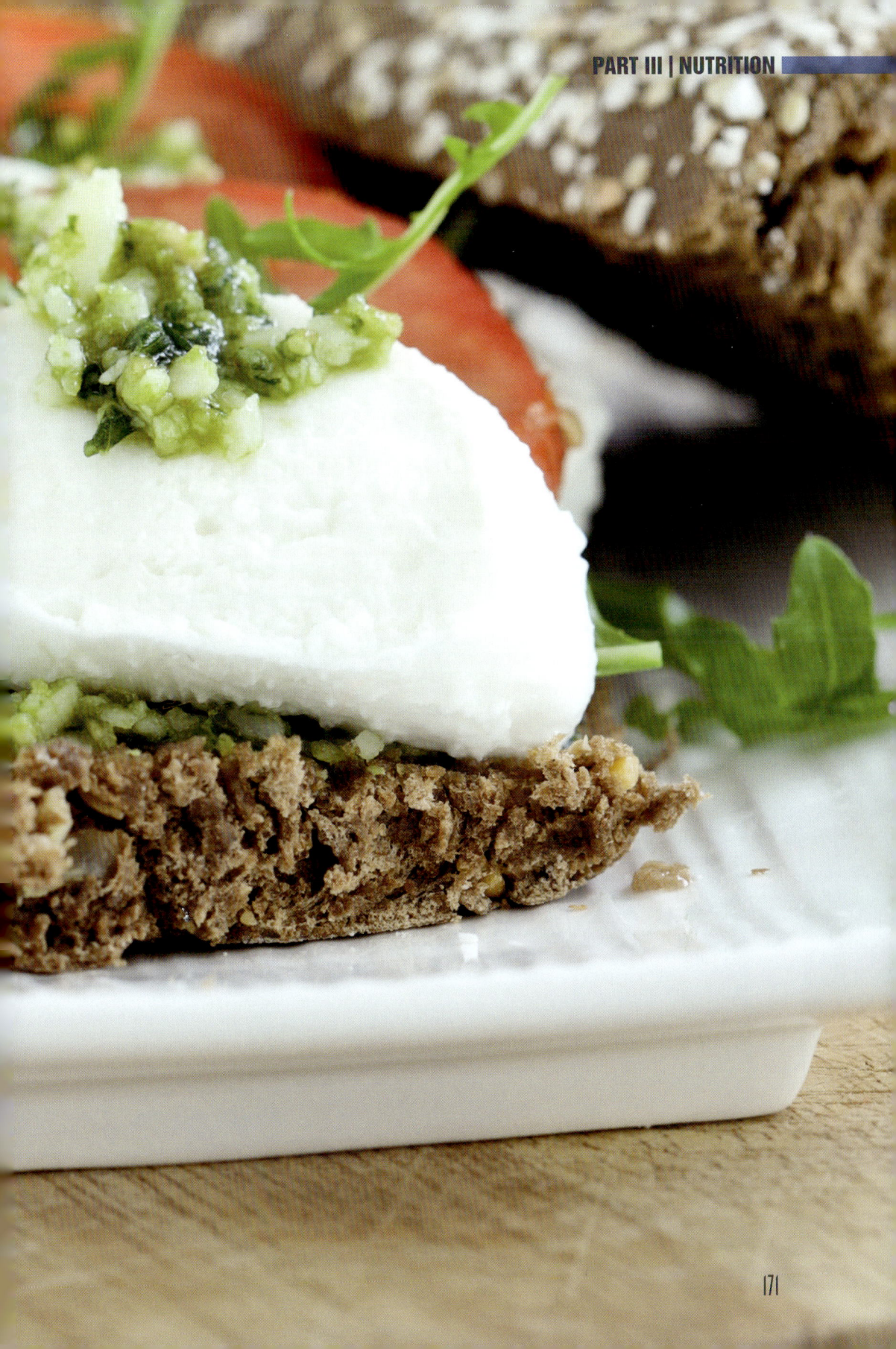

32 HOW TO KEEP ON TRACK

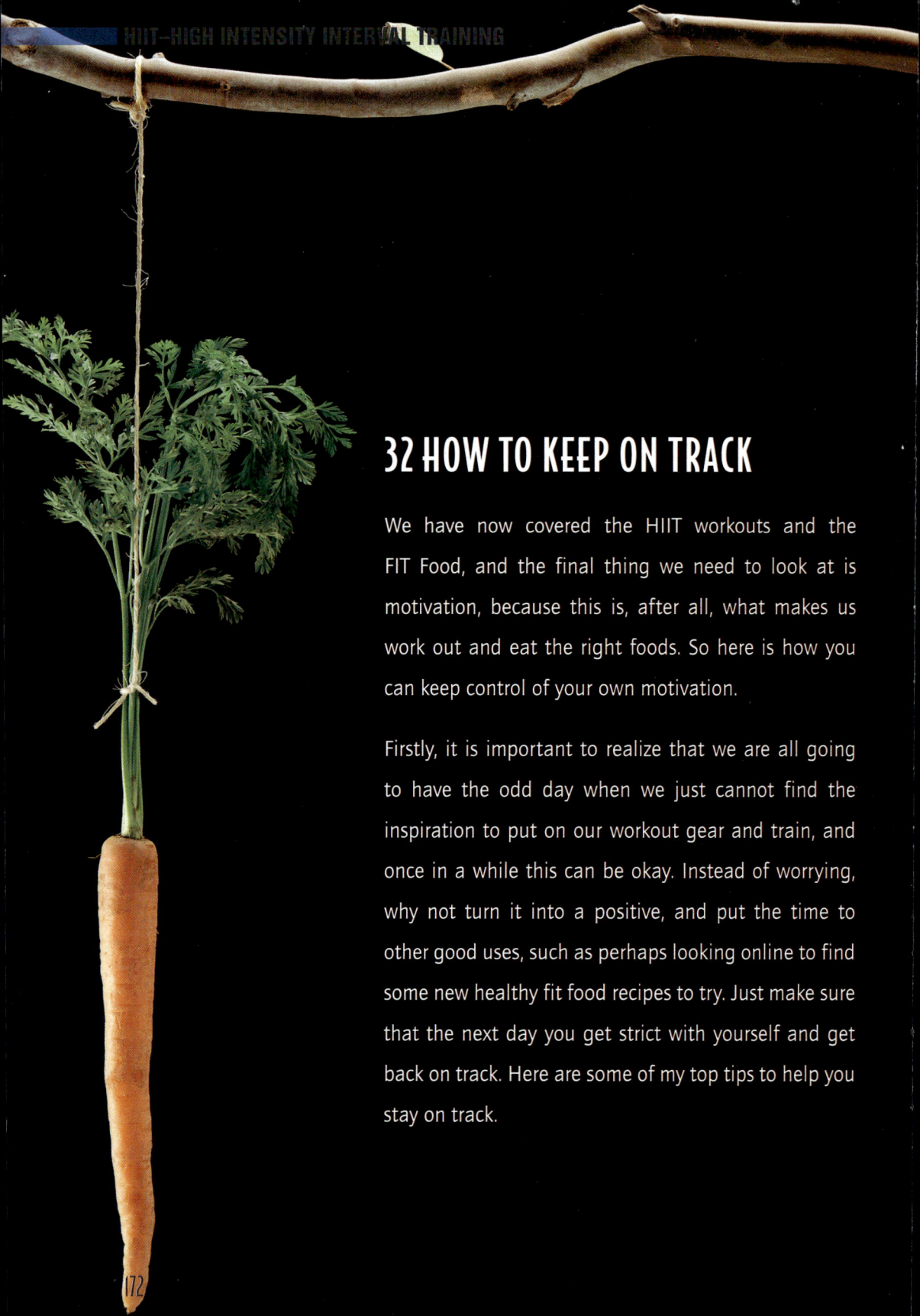

We have now covered the HIIT workouts and the FIT Food, and the final thing we need to look at is motivation, because this is, after all, what makes us work out and eat the right foods. So here is how you can keep control of your own motivation.

Firstly, it is important to realize that we are all going to have the odd day when we just cannot find the inspiration to put on our workout gear and train, and once in a while this can be okay. Instead of worrying, why not turn it into a positive, and put the time to other good uses, such as perhaps looking online to find some new healthy fit food recipes to try. Just make sure that the next day you get strict with yourself and get back on track. Here are some of my top tips to help you stay on track.

PART III | NUTRITION

TIP 1: GET SOCIAL

Use social media. (I am a big fan of this, because it is a great way to share with your friends and inspire others with your workouts and nutrition, and you in turn will feel inspired by others.) So get social with your new HIIT lifestyle, and do come and say hello to me on mine.

- Pinterest LWR FITNESS
- FaceBook LWR FITNESS
- Instagram @lucywyndhamread
- YouTube LWRFitnessChannel
- Twitter @lucywyndhamread

HIIT—HIGH INTENSITY INTERVAL TRAINING

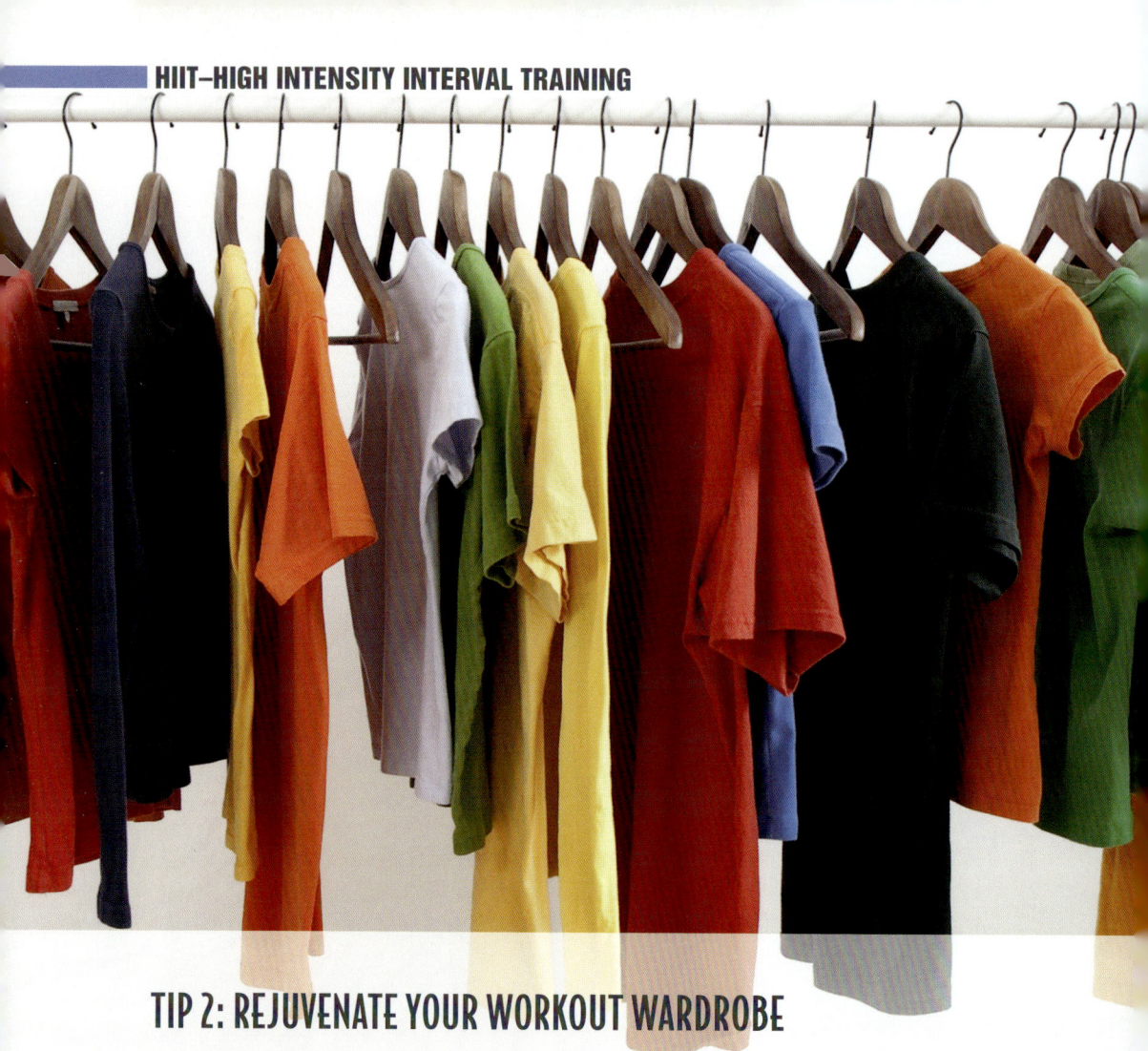

TIP 2: REJUVENATE YOUR WORKOUT WARDROBE

As you can see in my book, I have different outfits for every workout, and some in bright, vibrant colors. Purchasing some nice bright workout attire is a sound investment for your health.

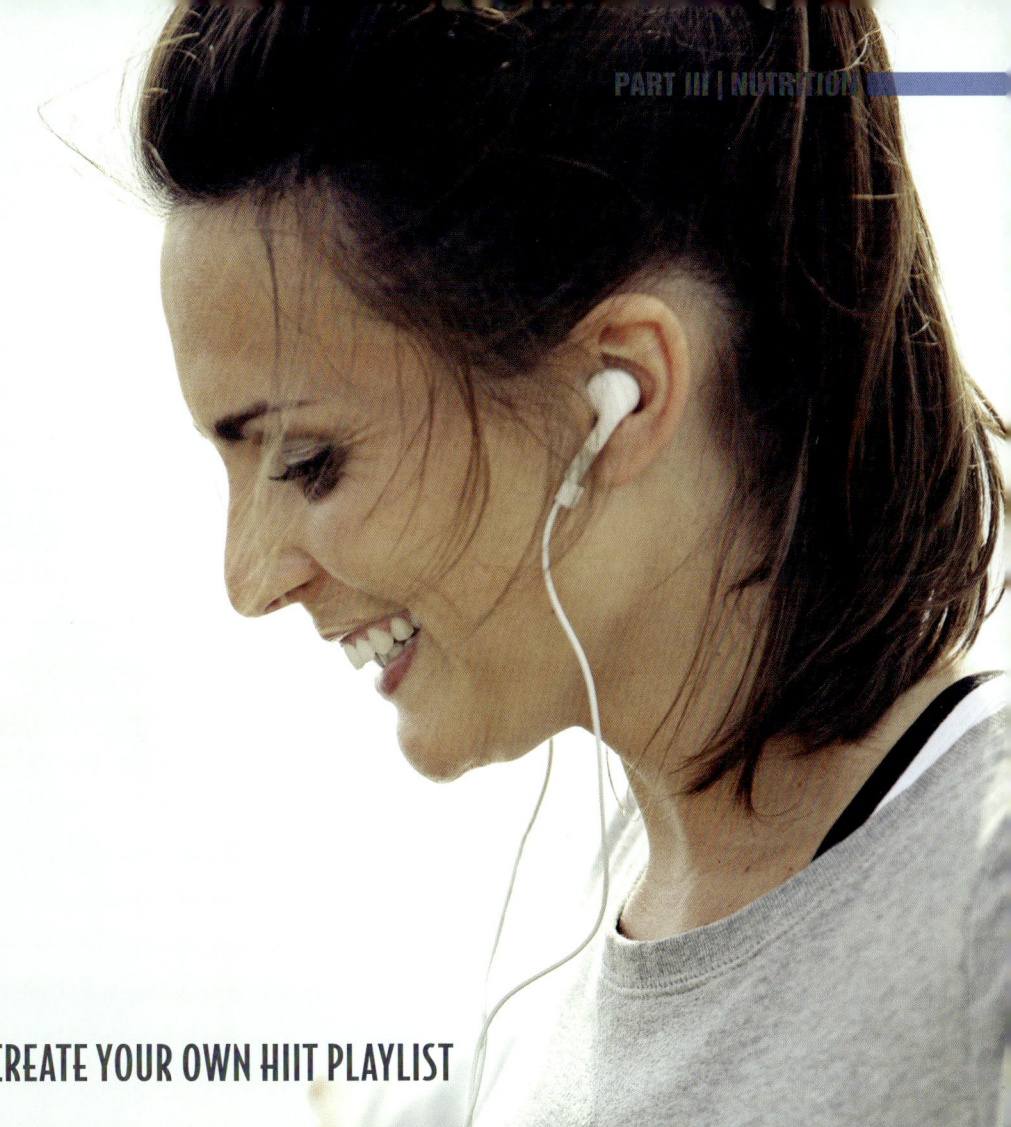

TIP 3: CREATE YOUR OWN HIIT PLAYLIST

Music is a great motivator in itself, so why not create some upbeat playlists for your favorite HIIT workouts. For the 4-minute HIIT workout, just one tune would probably do, whereas the walk HIIT workout will need several, so get creative with your tunes to add to your energy. And keep in mind that the faster the beat to the song, the harder we train.

HIIT—HIGH INTENSITY INTERVAL TRAINING

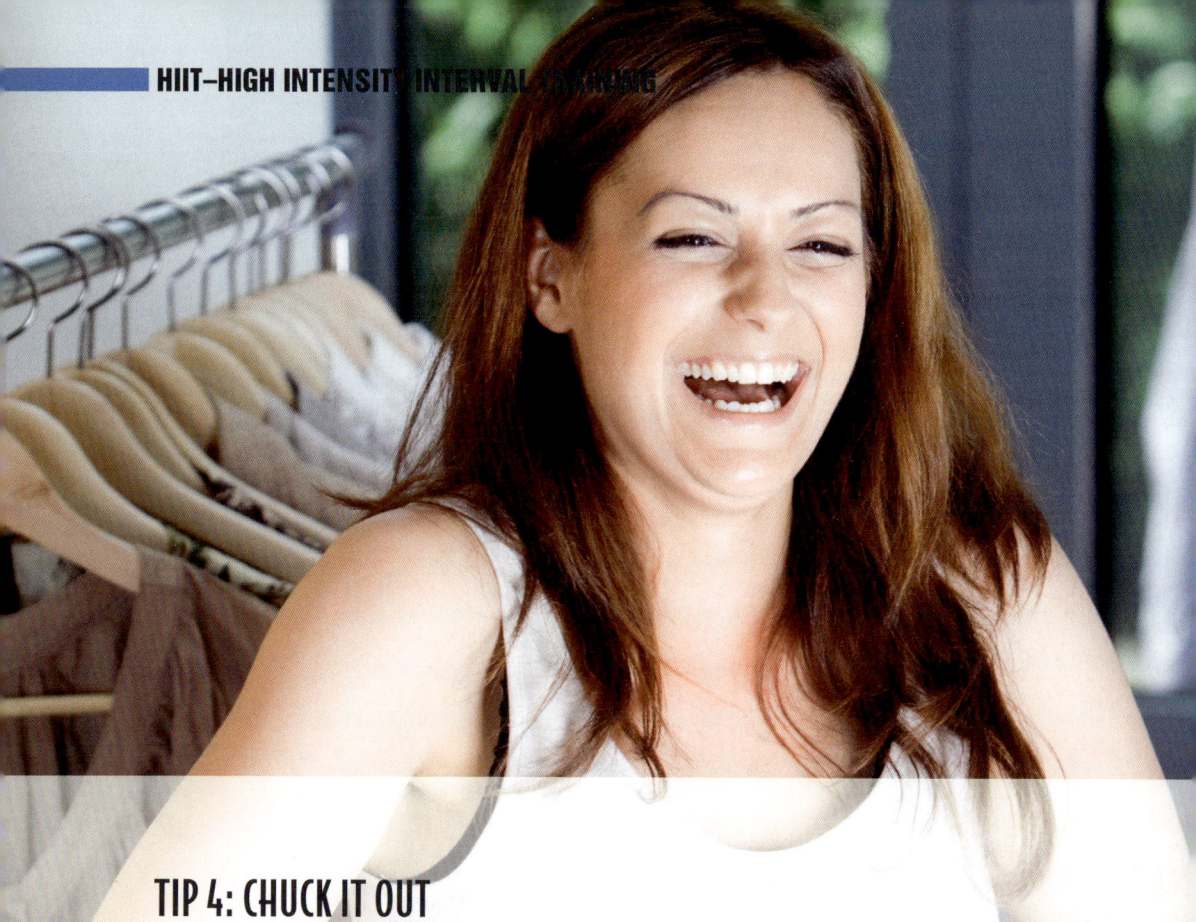

TIP 4: CHUCK IT OUT

If you are doing HIIT for weight loss, then once you've reached your target weight, throw out or give away every piece of clothing that no longer fits. The idea of having to buy a whole new wardrobe if you gain the weight back will serve as a strong incentive to maintain your new figure.

TIP 5: DETERMINATION AND DISCIPLINE

By this I mean simply just do it. After all, this book is full of super short workouts, so just don't let any excuses get in the way.

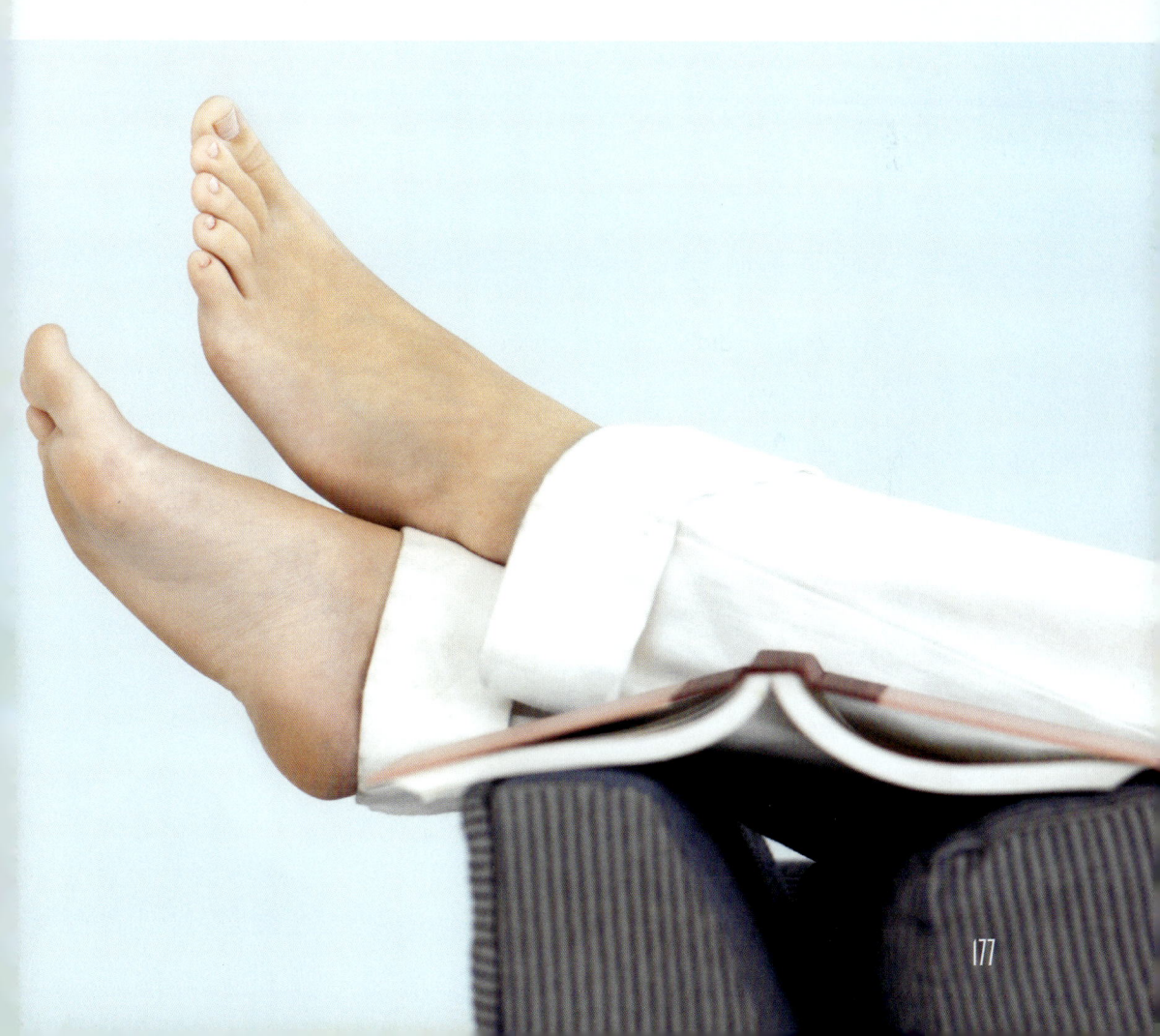

HIIT—HIGH INTENSITY INTERVAL TRAINING

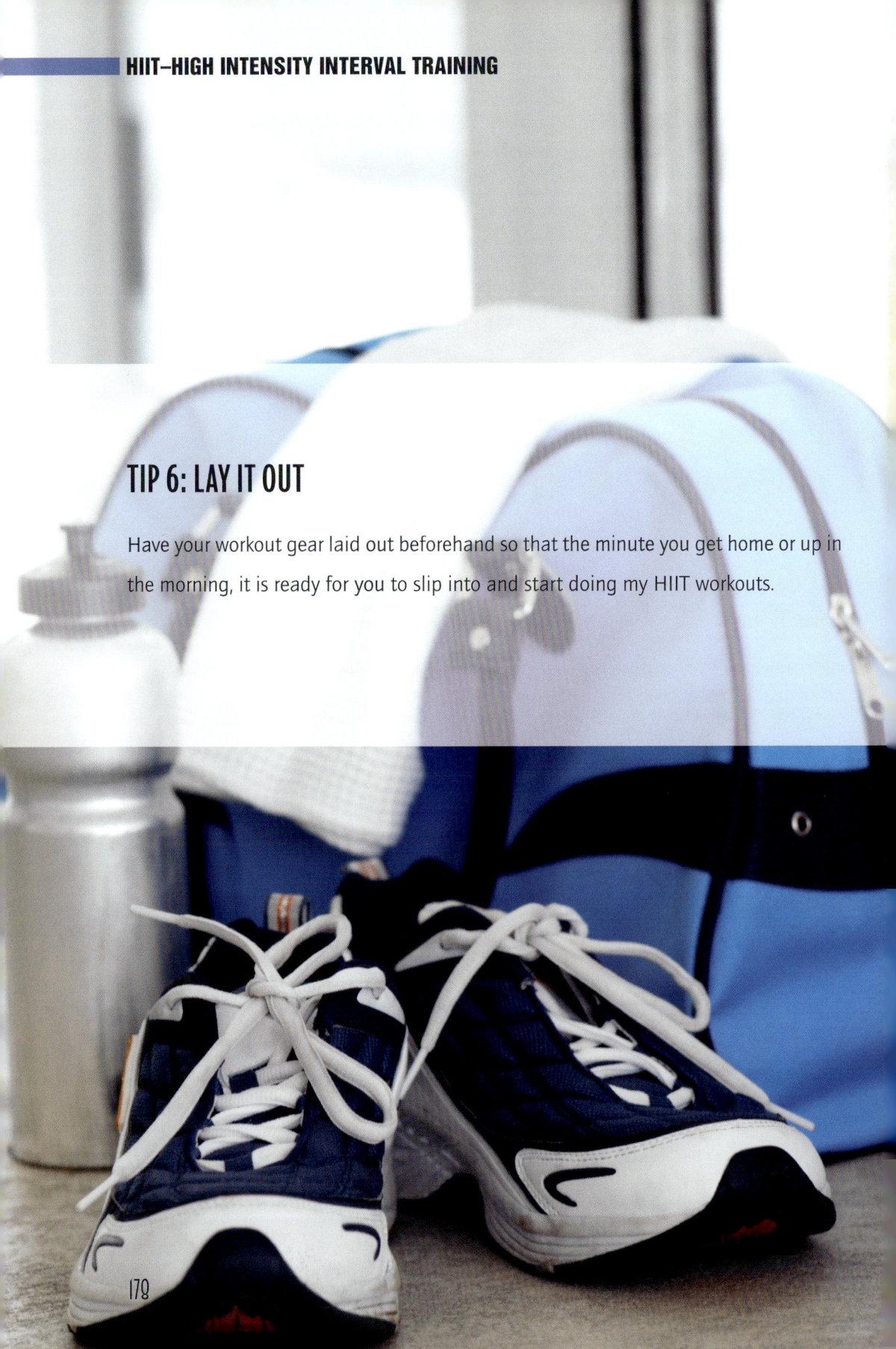

TIP 6: LAY IT OUT

Have your workout gear laid out beforehand so that the minute you get home or up in the morning, it is ready for you to slip into and start doing my HIIT workouts.

PART III | NUTRITION

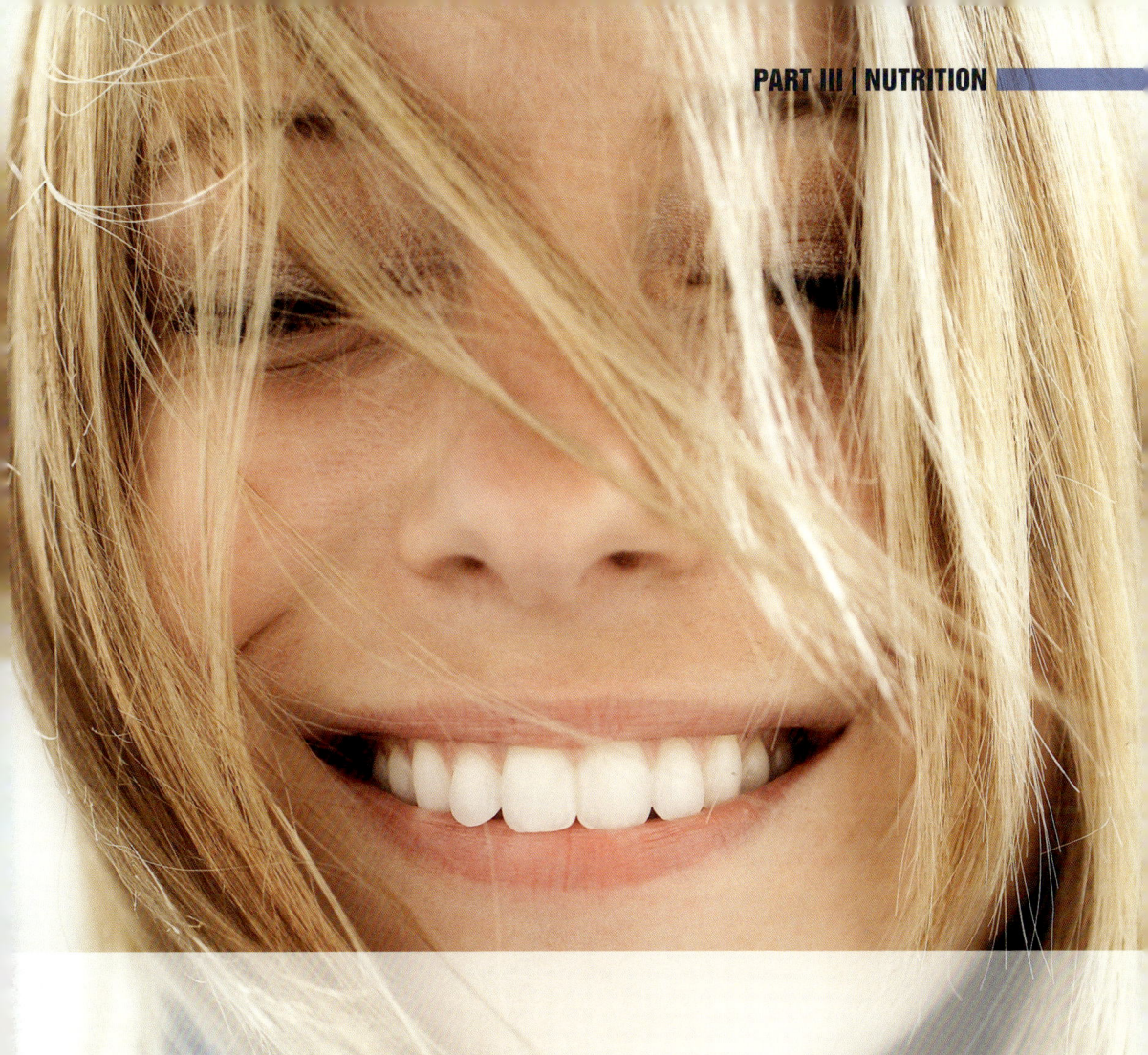

TIP 7: SEEING IS BELEVING

Visualize how you want to look and feel, and understand that you do have the power to be the fit, healthy, and strong person that you want to be. Just close those eyes and see how you will look if you stick to this easy and healthy and fit new lifestyle.

TIP 8: WHAT YOU GET

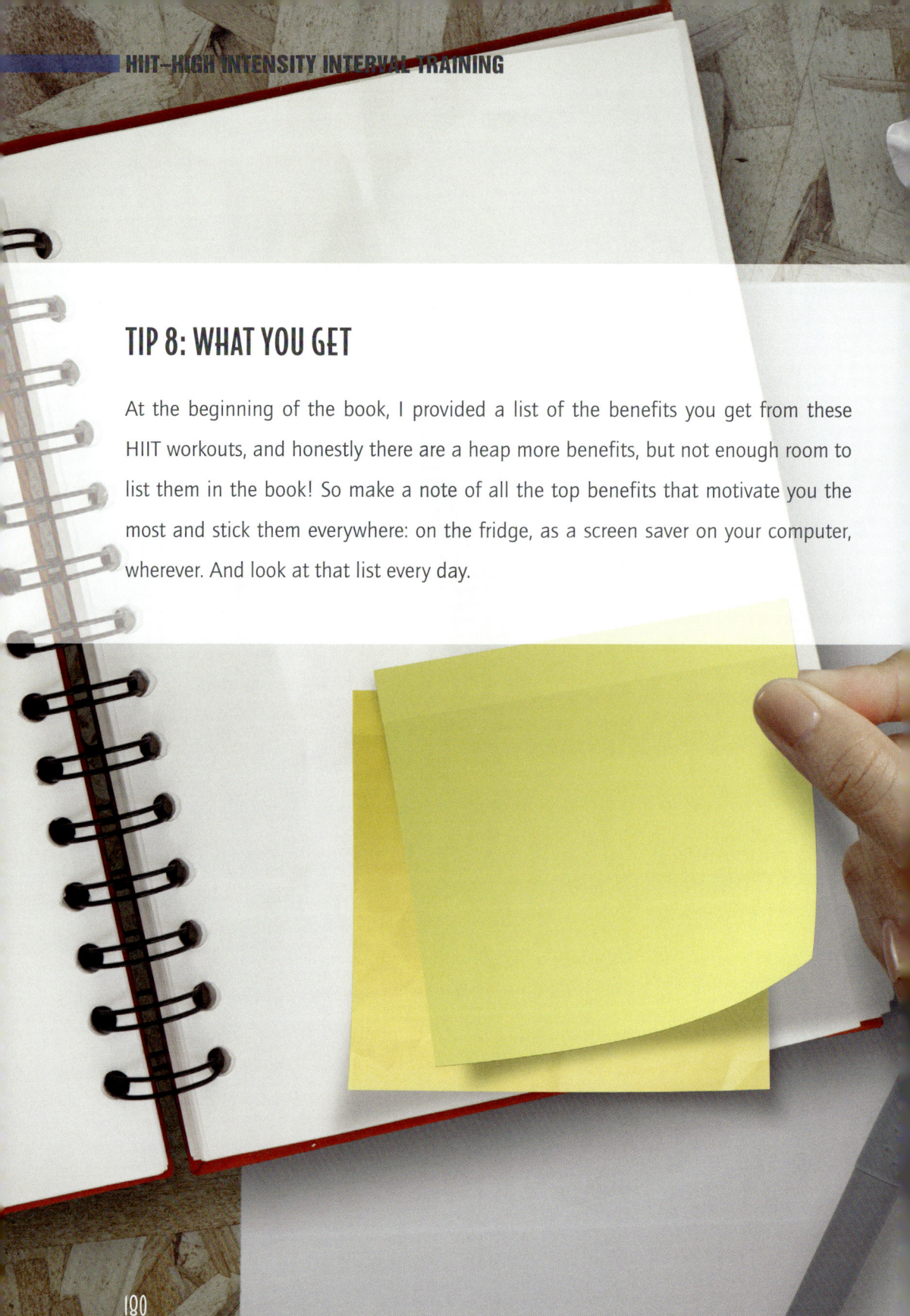

At the beginning of the book, I provided a list of the benefits you get from these HIIT workouts, and honestly there are a heap more benefits, but not enough room to list them in the book! So make a note of all the top benefits that motivate you the most and stick them everywhere: on the fridge, as a screen saver on your computer, wherever. And look at that list every day.

PART III | NUTRITION

And finally, once you are exercising regularly and eating a healthy diet, your body will always feel re-energised and fit and strong, and trust me, you will then have plenty of motivation, because you will love feeling this great.

For more tips on motivation, workouts, and recipes, come and visit my website: www.LWRFITNESS.com

I really hope you have enjoyed this book, and as exercise has been a big part of my life for the last 20 years, I can honestly say that HIIT training is my favorite workout of all time, because you can literally feel it working immediately. This method of training is one I have used on thousands of clients over the years, and they have all seen results quickly and been able to stick with these workouts because they are so easy to fit into any busy schedule.

Lucy

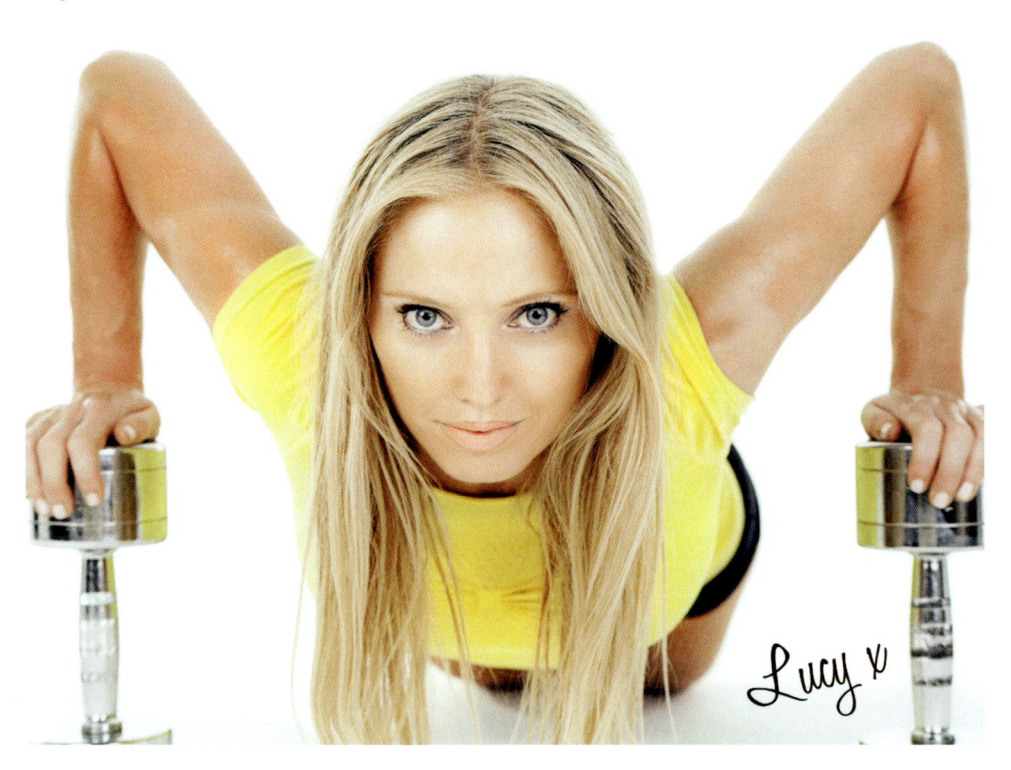

ACKNOWLEDGMENTS

There are a few people I would like to thank in helping bring this book to light, and that is my wonderful family and the two Michaels, who have been with me every step of the way; Hawthorns for the locations; Keith for all his help with editing and proofreading; Axl Stone for all his great photography; my fabulous stylist Michaela, who always gets it right and pulls it out of the bag every time; and finally all at Meyer and Meyer for making this into the best HIIT book.

CREDITS

Cover design:	Eva Feldmann, Aachen
Layout:	Andreas Reuel, Aachen
Typesetting:	Kerstin Quadflieg, Aachen
Photographs:	Axl Stone
	© Thinkstock/Stockbyte: pages 12-13, 176, 177, 178
	© Thinkstock/iStock: pages 22-23, 30-31, 34-35, 47-48, 147-148, 153-155, 158-159, 160-161, 162-163, 164-165, 166-167, 168-169, 170-171, 172, 174, 175, 180
	© Thinkstock/Wavebeak Media: page 43-44
	© Thinkstock/AbleSock.com: page 151-152
	© Thinkstock/Ingram Publishing: Paper on page 152
	© Thinkstock/Digital Vision: page 179
Copyediting:	Elizabeth Evans